Cannabis for Chronic Pain

A Nutritionist's Guide to Relief

Dr. Jade Hollis

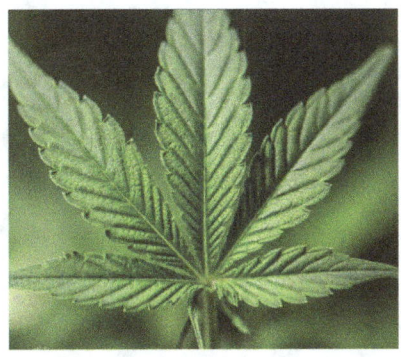

Cannabis for Chronic Pain: A Nutritionist's Guide to Relief

Cannabis for Chronic Pain: A Nutritionist's Guide to Relief

Copyright © 2024 by Dr. Jade Hollis

All rights reserved.

No part of this publication may be reproduced, distributed, or transmitted in any form or by any means, including photocopying, recording, or other electronic or mechanical methods, without the prior written permission of the author, except in the case of brief quotations embodied in critical reviews and certain other noncommercial uses permitted by copyright law. For permission requests, write to the publisher at the address below.

Published by Dr. Jade Hollis
Published via Amazon Kindle Direct Publishing

The content of this book is for informational purposes only and is not intended as a

Cannabis for Chronic Pain: A Nutritionist's Guide to Relief

substitute for professional medical advice, diagnosis, or treatment. Always seek the advice of your physician or other qualified health provider with any questions you may have regarding a medical condition.

Cover design by Dr. Jade Hollis

First Edition: December, 2024

Cannabis for Chronic Pain: A Nutritionist's Guide to Relief

To those who endure chronic pain with courage and resilience,
May this guide bring you hope, relief, and empowerment on your journey to wellness.

And to the researchers, practitioners, and pioneers in cannabis and nutrition therapy. Your dedication inspires a brighter, healthier future for us all.

With gratitude,
Dr. Jade Hollis

Cannabis for Chronic Pain: A Nutritionist's Guide to Relief

CONTENTS

Part 1: Foundations of Cannabis and Chronic Pain — 16

1.1: Introduction to Cannabis and Chronic Pain — 16

Overview of the Endocannabinoid System — 17
- Components of the ECS — 17
- The ECS and Pain Regulation — 19
- Cannabis and the ECS — 20

Prevalence and Impact of Chronic Pain — 22
- Defining Chronic Pain — 22
- Epidemiology of Chronic Pain — 22
- Economic and Social Impact — 23
- Limitations of Conventional Pain Management — 24

Rationale for Using Cannabis for Chronic Pain Management — 24
- Cannabis as a Multi-Target Therapy — 25
- Scientific Evidence Supporting Cannabis Use — 26
- Advantages of Cannabis Over Traditional Therapies — 27

Practical Applications for Cannabis in Chronic Pain Management — 28
- Integrative Approaches — 28
- Patient-Centered Care — 28
- Barriers and Challenges — 29

1.2: The Science of Cannabis and Pain Relief — 31

Cannabis for Chronic Pain: A Nutritionist's Guide to Relief

Mechanisms of Cannabis-Induced Pain Relief — 31
1. Modulation of the Endocannabinoid System — 32
2. Anti-Inflammatory Effects — 33
3. Desensitization of Pain Pathways — 34
4. Neuromodulation — 34
5. Psychotropic Effects and Pain Perception — 35

THC, CBD, and Other Cannabinoids: Roles in Pain Management — 35
1. THC (Δ9-Tetrahydrocannabinol) — 36
2. CBD (Cannabidiol) — 37
3. Other Cannabinoids — 38

Current Research on Cannabis and Pain Relief — 39
1. Clinical Evidence — 39
2. Comparative Studies with Conventional Treatments — 40
3. Preclinical Studies — 41
4. Limitations and Challenges in Research — 42

Practical Applications of Cannabis for Pain Relief — 43
1. Delivery Methods — 43
2. Dosing Strategies — 43
3. Combining Cannabinoids — 44

1.3: Nutrition and Chronic Pain: The Basics — 46

The Impact of Nutrition on Chronic Pain — 47

Cannabis for Chronic Pain: A Nutritionist's Guide to Relief

    1. The Inflammatory Connection   47
    2. Gut Health and Pain Modulation   48
    3. Blood Sugar Regulation and Pain   49

Key Nutrients and Dietary Patterns for Pain Management   50
    1. Anti-Inflammatory Nutrients   50
    2. Pain-Reducing Dietary Patterns   52

Introduction to the Concept of "Food as Medicine"   53
    1. Historical Context   54
    2. Modern Applications   54

Practical Applications for Chronic Pain Management   55
    1. Creating a Pain-Relief Diet Plan   56
    2. Lifestyle Integration   56

Current Research and Future Directions   57
    1. Evidence from Clinical Studies   57
    2. Emerging Areas of Study   58

Part 2: Cannabis and Nutrition for Chronic Pain Management   60

2.1: Cannabis and Omega-3 Fatty Acids: A Powerful Pain-Relieving Combination   60

The Role of Omega-3 Fatty Acids in Pain Management   63
    1. Understanding Omega-3 Fatty Acids   63
    2. Mechanisms of Pain Relief   64
    3. Clinical Evidence   65

Cannabis and Omega-3 Fatty Acids: Mechanistic Interactions   66

Cannabis for Chronic Pain: A Nutritionist's Guide to Relief

    1. The Endocannabinoid System and Omega-3s   66

    2. Cannabis Synergy with Omega-3s   67

Current Research on Cannabis and Omega-3s in Pain Relief   68

    1. Preclinical Studies   69

    2. Clinical Studies   69

    3. Ongoing Research Areas   70

Practical Applications: Integrating Cannabis and Omega-3s for Pain Relief 71

    1. Dietary Recommendations   71

    2. Cannabis Administration   72

    3. Combined Therapy Protocol   72

2.2: The Impact of Cannabis on Gut Health and Chronic Pain   74

The Gut-Brain Axis and Its Role in Chronic Pain   75

    1. Anatomy and Function of the Gut-Brain Axis   75

    2. Gut-Related Pain Pathways   76

    3. Clinical Evidence of Gut-Brain Axis in Chronic Pain   77

How Cannabis Affects Gut Health and Chronic Pain   78

    1. The Endocannabinoid System in the Gut   78

    2. Cannabis and Inflammation in the Gut 79

    3. Cannabis and Gut Motility   79

    4. Clinical Evidence: Cannabis for Gut-Related Chronic Pain   80

Nutritional Strategies for Promoting Gut Health and Cannabis Efficacy — 81
- 1. The Role of Diet in Gut Health — 81
- 2. Optimizing Cannabis Efficacy Through Nutrition — 82
- 3. Diet Plans for Gut and Pain Management — 83

Practical Applications and Case Studies — 84
- 1. Integrating Cannabis and Gut-Healthy Nutrition — 84
- 2. Case Study: IBS and Cannabis — 84
- 3. Case Study: Fibromyalgia with Gut Dysbiosis — 85

2.3: Cannabis, Magnesium, and Muscle Relaxation: A Trio for Pain Relief — 87

1. The Role of Magnesium in Muscle Relaxation and Pain Management — 90
- 1.1. Magnesium and Muscle Function — 90
- 1.2. Magnesium's Role in Pain Modulation — 91
- 1.3. Research Supporting Magnesium's Role in Pain Relief — 93

2. How Cannabis and Magnesium Interact to Enhance Pain Relief — 94
- 2.1. Cannabis and the Endocannabinoid System (ECS) — 94
- 2.2. The Synergy Between Magnesium and Cannabis — 96
- 2.3. Research on Cannabis and Magnesium Interaction — 97

3. Nutritional Strategies for Optimizing

Magnesium Levels and Cannabis Efficacy — 98
- 3.1. Dietary Sources of Magnesium — 99
- 3.2. Magnesium Supplementation — 100
- 3.3. Optimizing Cannabis Use for Pain Relief — 101
- 3.4. Combining Magnesium and Cannabis in Treatment Plans — 102

Part 3: Putting it All Together - A Comprehensive Approach to Cannabis and Nutrition for Chronic Pain — 104

3.1: Creating a Personalized Cannabis and Nutrition Plan for Chronic Pain — 104

1. Assessing Individual Needs and Health Status — 107
- 1.1. Comprehensive Health Assessment — 107
- 1.2. Pain Profile and Type of Pain — 109
- 1.3. Personal Preferences and Treatment Goals — 110

2. Setting Goals and Developing a Treatment Plan — 111
- 2.1. Defining Treatment Goals — 112
- 2.2. Developing a Personalized Cannabis Plan — 113
- 2.3. Nutritional Strategies to Support Pain Relief — 115
- 2.4. Integrating Cannabis and Nutrition — 117

3. Monitoring Progress and Adjusting the Plan — 118
- 3.1. Regular Check-ins and Pain

- Tracking 118
- 3.2. Adjusting Dosage and Delivery Methods 119
- 3.3. Adjusting Nutritional Strategies 120
- 3.4. Feedback Loop and Continuous Improvement 120

3.2: Cannabis and Nutrition Interactions: What to Watch Out For 122

1. Potential Interactions Between Cannabis and Medications 125
- 1.1. Role of Cytochrome P450 Enzymes 125
- 1.2. Common Medications Affected by Cannabis 126
- 1.3. Risk Factors for Adverse Drug-Cannabis Interactions 127

2. Nutritional Considerations for Minimizing Adverse Effects 128
- 2.1. Enhancing Liver Function 129
- 2.2. Addressing Nutritional Deficiencies 130
- 2.3. Mitigating Side Effects of Cannabis 131
- 2.4. Timing Meals and Cannabis Use 131

3. Strategies for Mitigating Potential Interactions 132
- 3.1. Collaborative Care 132
- 3.2. Personalizing Cannabis Dosing 133
- 3.3. Regular Monitoring and Adjustments 134
- 3.4. Education and Awareness 134

    3.5. Alternative Therapies   135

3.3: Overcoming Challenges and Staying Motivated: A Guide for Patients and Practitioners   138

    1. Common Challenges in Cannabis and Nutrition Therapy   138

        1.1. Challenges for Patients   139

        1.2. Challenges for Practitioners   141

    2. Strategies for Overcoming Challenges and Staying Motivated   142

        2.1. For Patients   143

        2.2. For Practitioners   145

    3. Resources for Further Support and Guidance   147

        3.1. For Patients   147

        3.2. For Practitioners   148

Part 4: Case Studies and Future Directions   150

4.1: Real-Life Examples of Cannabis and Nutrition Therapy for Chronic Pain   151

    1. Case Study 1: Managing Fibromyalgia with Cannabis and an Anti-Inflammatory Diet   153

        Background   153

        Intervention   153

        Outcomes   154

        Key Takeaways   154

    2. Case Study 2: Alleviating Osteoarthritis Pain with Cannabis and Collagen Supplementation   155

        Background   155

        Intervention   156

Outcomes ... 156
Key Takeaways ... 157

3. Case Study 3: Treating Migraine Pain with Cannabis and Magnesium Optimization ... 157

Background ... 157
Intervention ... 158
Outcomes ... 159
Key Takeaways ... 159

4. Lessons Learned from Case Studies ... 160

5. Practical Applications for Patients and Practitioners ... 161

For Patients ... 161
For Practitioners ... 162

4.2: The Future of Cannabis and Nutrition Research: Emerging Trends and Opportunities ... 162

1. Overview of Current Research Gaps ... 164

1.1. Lack of Large-Scale, Longitudinal Studies ... 165
1.2. Insufficient Focus on Individual Variability ... 166
1.3. Interactions Between Cannabis and Nutrients ... 167
1.4. Limited Research on Special Populations ... 167

2. Emerging Trends in Cannabis and Nutrition Research ... 168

2.1. Integration of Personalized Medicine ... 168

2.2. The Role of the Microbiome 168
2.3. Advances in Cannabinoid Delivery Systems 169
2.4. Exploration of Terpenes and Flavonoids 170
2.5. Multi-Modal Therapies 170

3. Opportunities in Cannabis and Nutrition Research 171

3.1. Cross-Disciplinary Collaborations 171
3.2. Use of Artificial Intelligence (AI) and Machine Learning 171
3.3. Expanding the Scope of Cannabinoid Research 172
3.4. Ethical and Regulatory Considerations 172

4. Implications for Clinical Practice and Patient Care 173

4.1. Enhanced Patient Education 173
4.2. Evidence-Based Protocols 173
4.3. Focus on Holistic Care 173

4.3: Conclusion and Final Thoughts 174

1. Recap of Key Takeaways 175

1.1. The Science Behind Cannabis and Pain Management 175
1.2. Nutrition's Role in Chronic Pain Management 176
1.3. Cannabis and Nutrition: A Synergistic Approach 177
1.4. Practical Strategies for Implementation 178

2. Final Thoughts on the Potential of

Cannabis for Chronic Pain: A Nutritionist's Guide to Relief

Cannabis and Nutrition Therapy — 179
- 2.1. A Paradigm Shift in Chronic Pain Management — 179
- 2.2. Bridging the Gaps in Knowledge and Access — 179
- 2.3. Holistic Care for Complex Conditions — 180

3. Encouragement for Further Exploration and Discovery — 181
- 3.1. For Practitioners — 181
- 3.2. For Patients — 181
- 3.3. For Researchers and Innovators — 182

4. Practical Implications and Vision for the Future — 182
- 4.1. Building Comprehensive Care Models — 183
- 4.2. A Sustainable Approach to Health — 183
- 4.3. Expanding the Therapeutic Toolbox — 183

Cannabis for Chronic Pain: A Nutritionist's Guide to Relief

Part 1: Foundations of Cannabis and Chronic Pain

1.1: Introduction to Cannabis and Chronic Pain

Chronic pain is a pervasive health challenge affecting millions globally. With its multifaceted origins and significant impact on quality of life, effective management often requires an integrative approach. Cannabis has emerged as a promising alternative or adjunctive therapy, particularly for individuals who have not found relief through conventional treatments. This chapter explores the foundational elements connecting cannabis and chronic pain management, beginning with the endocannabinoid system (ECS), the prevalence and impact of chronic pain, and the

Cannabis for Chronic Pain: A Nutritionist's Guide to Relief

rationale for using cannabis to address this condition.

Overview of the Endocannabinoid System

The endocannabinoid system (ECS) is a critical regulatory network responsible for maintaining homeostasis within the body. Its discovery has revolutionized our understanding of various physiological processes, particularly in relation to pain perception, inflammation, and immune response.

Components of the ECS

1. Endocannabinoids

Lipid-based neurotransmitters synthesized on demand by the body.

The two primary endocannabinoids are:

- **Anandamide (AEA):** Often called the "bliss molecule," it plays a role in regulating mood, appetite, and pain.

- **2-Arachidonoylglycerol (2-AG):** Involved in managing inflammation and modulating pain.

2. Cannabinoid Receptors

The ECS operates through cannabinoid receptors located throughout the body:

- **CB1 Receptors:** Predominantly found in the brain and central nervous system; associated with pain modulation, memory, and mood.

- **CB2 Receptors:** Primarily located in immune cells and peripheral tissues; involved in managing inflammation and immune responses.

3. Enzymes

Enzymes regulate the breakdown of endocannabinoids:

- **Fatty Acid Amide Hydrolase (FAAH):** Degrades anandamide.
- **Monoacylglycerol Lipase (MAGL):** Breaks down 2-AG.

The ECS and Pain Regulation

- The ECS is integral to nociception, the process by which pain signals are transmitted and processed.
- When activated, cannabinoid receptors modulate the release of neurotransmitters, dampening the perception of pain and reducing inflammation.
- Dysregulation of the ECS has been linked to various chronic pain conditions, including fibromyalgia, arthritis, and neuropathic pain.

Cannabis for Chronic Pain: A Nutritionist's Guide to Relief

Cannabis and the ECS

Phytocannabinoids from the cannabis plant, such as THC and CBD, mimic endocannabinoids and interact with the ECS to provide therapeutic effects:

 - **THC (Δ9-Tetrahydrocannabinol):** Binds to CB1 and CB2 receptors, modulating pain and inducing euphoria.

 - **CBD (Cannabidiol):** Indirectly influences the ECS by inhibiting FAAH and enhancing anandamide levels, offering anti-inflammatory and analgesic effects.

Cannabis for Chronic Pain: A Nutritionist's Guide to Relief

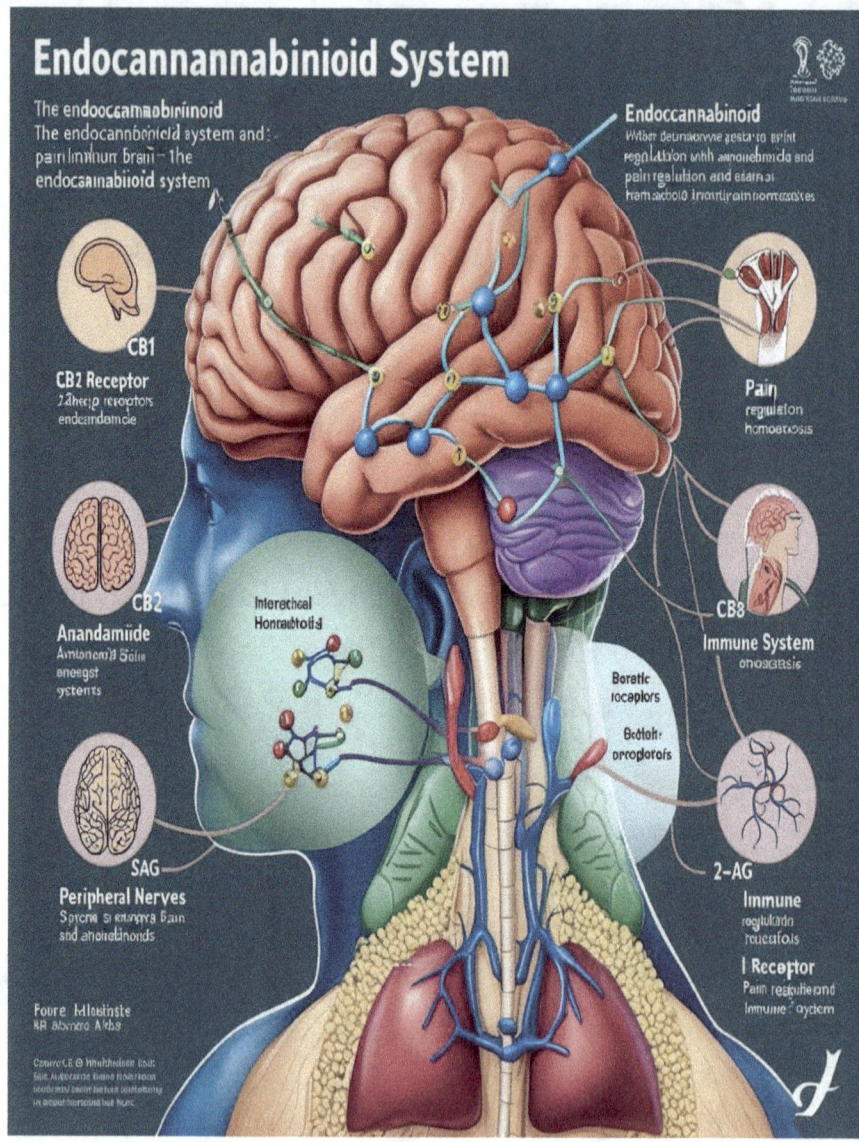

The Endocannabinoid System in Action

Prevalence and Impact of Chronic Pain

Defining Chronic Pain

Chronic pain is pain that persists for longer than three to six months, often beyond the typical healing period of an injury or illness. It is characterized by its multifactorial nature, encompassing physical, psychological, and social dimensions.

Epidemiology of Chronic Pain

- **Global Prevalence:**
  Chronic pain affects approximately 20-30% of the global population, with significant variations based on age, gender, and region.
- **United States Statistics:**
  Nearly 50 million adults in the U.S. experience chronic pain, with 19.6 million

reporting high-impact chronic pain that interferes with daily activities.

Common conditions include arthritis, back pain, migraines, and neuropathic pain.

Economic and Social Impact

1. Healthcare Costs:
   - Chronic pain accounts for billions in direct medical expenses annually.
   - Indirect costs include lost productivity and absenteeism.

2. Psychological Burden:
   - Individuals with chronic pain are more likely to experience depression, anxiety, and social isolation.

3. Impact on Quality of Life:
   - Chronic pain impairs physical function, limits mobility, and reduces overall well-being.

Cannabis for Chronic Pain: A Nutritionist's Guide to Relief

Limitations of Conventional Pain Management

- Over-reliance on opioids has led to significant public health challenges, including addiction and overdose.
- Nonsteroidal anti-inflammatory drugs (NSAIDs) may cause gastrointestinal, cardiovascular, and renal side effects with prolonged use.
- Many patients seek alternative therapies, including cannabis, due to the inadequacy or adverse effects of traditional treatments.

Rationale for Using Cannabis for Chronic Pain Management

Cannabis for Chronic Pain: A Nutritionist's Guide to Relief

Cannabis offers a multifaceted approach to managing chronic pain, addressing both the sensory and emotional aspects of pain. Its integration into pain management strategies is supported by emerging scientific evidence and patient-reported outcomes.

Cannabis as a Multi-Target Therapy

- Cannabis is particularly effective for chronic pain due to its ability to influence multiple pathways simultaneously:
  - Modulation of **nociceptive signals** through CB1 receptor activation.
  - Reduction of **inflammation** via CB2 receptor engagement.
  - Enhancement of **mood** and reduction of pain-related distress through indirect effects on serotonin and dopamine systems.

Cannabis for Chronic Pain: A Nutritionist's Guide to Relief

Scientific Evidence Supporting Cannabis Use

1. Clinical Trials and Systematic Reviews

Studies indicate that cannabis and cannabinoids are effective for various types of chronic pain, including:

- **Neuropathic Pain**: Cannabis has been shown to reduce pain intensity and improve sleep quality in patients with conditions like multiple sclerosis.

- **Cancer Pain:** Adjunctive use of cannabis reduces opioid requirements and enhances pain relief.

- **Arthritis Pain:** Topical and oral cannabis formulations alleviate joint pain and inflammation.

2. Patient-Reported Outcomes

Surveys and observational studies highlight that patients report significant improvements in pain, sleep, and overall quality of life with cannabis use.

Cannabis for Chronic Pain: A Nutritionist's Guide to Relief

Advantages of Cannabis Over Traditional Therapies

- **Reduced Risk of Dependence**: Unlike opioids, cannabis has a lower potential for addiction and withdrawal symptoms.
- **Fewer Side Effects**: Common side effects like dry mouth and mild dizziness are less severe compared to the gastrointestinal or cardiovascular risks of NSAIDs.
- **Non-Invasive Application**: Cannabis can be administered in various forms, including oils, tinctures, topicals, and edibles, allowing personalized treatment plans.

Practical Applications for Cannabis in Chronic Pain Management

Integrative Approaches

Cannabis is most effective when used as part of a holistic pain management plan that includes:
- **Nutrition**: Incorporating anti-inflammatory diets to complement cannabis's effects.
- **Physical Therapy**: Addressing musculoskeletal imbalances that contribute to pain.
- **Mindfulness Practices**: Utilizing meditation and cognitive behavioral therapy (CBT) to enhance pain coping mechanisms.

Patient-Centered Care

- **Personalized Dosing**: The ideal cannabis regimen varies based on the individual's condition, ECS profile, and tolerance.
- **Education**: Patients and healthcare providers must understand cannabis's benefits, risks, and legal considerations.

Barriers and Challenges

- **Legal Restrictions**: Despite increasing legalization, access to medical cannabis remains limited in some regions.
- **Stigma**: Negative perceptions about cannabis use may deter patients from considering it as a viable option.
- **Knowledge Gaps**: Many healthcare professionals lack formal training on cannabis, underscoring the need for education and advocacy.

Cannabis for Chronic Pain: A Nutritionist's Guide to Relief

Cannabis represents a transformative tool in chronic pain management, grounded in its interaction with the ECS and supported by growing scientific evidence. By addressing both physical and emotional aspects of pain, cannabis offers a promising alternative to traditional therapies. As research continues to evolve, its integration into comprehensive pain management strategies has the potential to improve outcomes and enhance quality of life for millions of patients.

In subsequent chapters, we will delve deeper into the specific mechanisms of cannabis-induced pain relief, as well as its interplay with nutritional strategies for optimal therapeutic outcomes.

1.2: The Science of Cannabis and Pain Relief

Cannabis has been used for centuries as a natural remedy for pain relief. Recent advances in scientific research have provided a deeper understanding of how cannabis and its compounds alleviate pain. This chapter delves into the mechanisms of cannabis-induced pain relief, explores the specific roles of cannabinoids like THC and CBD, and reviews current research to elucidate the potential and limitations of cannabis in pain management.

Mechanisms of Cannabis-Induced Pain Relief

Cannabis for Chronic Pain: A Nutritionist's Guide to Relief

Cannabis relieves pain through its interaction with the endocannabinoid system (ECS) and other physiological pathways. These mechanisms address both nociceptive (physical) and neuropathic (nerve-related) pain, offering a comprehensive approach to pain management.

1. Modulation of the Endocannabinoid System

1. Cannabinoid Receptors (CB1 and CB2):
   - **CB1 Receptors**: Located predominantly in the brain and central nervous system, CB1 receptors regulate the transmission of pain signals. Activation reduces the release of excitatory neurotransmitters, dampening pain perception.
   - **CB2 Receptors**: Found in immune cells and peripheral tissues, CB2 receptors help

control inflammation, a common contributor to chronic pain.

2. Endocannabinoid Regulation:

- Cannabis compounds enhance the levels of endogenous cannabinoids like anandamide by inhibiting enzymes such as FAAH (Fatty Acid Amide Hydrolase).
- This amplification strengthens the body's natural pain-relief processes.

2. Anti-Inflammatory Effects

Cannabinoids reduce the production of pro-inflammatory cytokines, molecules involved in chronic inflammation. This action is particularly beneficial for conditions like arthritis and autoimmune diseases, where inflammation exacerbates pain.

3. Desensitization of Pain Pathways

TRPV1 (Transient Receptor Potential Vanilloid 1) Channels:
 - Cannabinoids desensitize these receptors, which are involved in detecting heat, acidity, and pain.
 - Desensitization results in reduced sensitivity to painful stimuli.

- Glycine Receptors:
 - THC activates glycine receptors in the spinal cord, inhibiting pain transmission to the brain.

4. Neuromodulation

Cannabinoids influence various neurotransmitter systems:
- Dopaminergic System: Enhances mood and reduces pain perception by increasing dopamine levels.

- Serotonergic System: Modulates serotonin receptors, contributing to both pain relief and mood stabilization.

5. Psychotropic Effects and Pain Perception

- Cannabis, particularly THC, alters the emotional experience of pain by activating brain regions associated with reward and pleasure.
- This psychotropic effect can shift the focus away from pain, improving overall coping mechanisms.

THC, CBD, and Other Cannabinoids: Roles in Pain Management

Cannabis for Chronic Pain: A Nutritionist's Guide to Relief

The cannabis plant contains over 100 cannabinoids, each with distinct roles in pain relief. Among these, THC and CBD are the most researched and widely used, but other minor cannabinoids also show therapeutic potential.

1. THC (Δ9-Tetrahydrocannabinol)

1. Mechanism of Action:
 - THC binds directly to CB1 receptors in the brain, altering pain signaling and perception.
 - It also binds to CB2 receptors, reducing inflammation.

2. Therapeutic Benefits:
 - Effective for both nociceptive and neuropathic pain.
 - Particularly useful for conditions like cancer pain, multiple sclerosis, and spinal cord injuries.

3. Limitations and Side Effects:
   - Psychoactive effects such as euphoria, dizziness, and potential anxiety.
   - Risk of dependence with long-term use.

2. CBD (Cannabidiol)

1. Mechanism of Action:
   - CBD does not bind directly to CB1 or CB2 receptors. Instead, it modulates receptor activity and enhances the effects of endogenous cannabinoids.
   - Influences non-cannabinoid receptors like TRPV1 and serotonin receptors.

2. Therapeutic Benefits:
   - Reduces inflammation and neuropathic pain without causing psychoactive effects.
   - Synergistic effects with THC, enhancing pain relief while mitigating THC's side effects.

3. Applications:
- Effective for conditions such as arthritis, fibromyalgia, and diabetic neuropathy.

3. Other Cannabinoids

1. CBG (Cannabigerol):
- Anti-inflammatory properties with potential for treating inflammatory bowel disease (IBD) and chronic pain.

2. CBN (Cannabinol):
- Mildly psychoactive, promotes relaxation, and may help with pain-related insomnia.

3. THCV (Tetrahydrocannabivarin):
- Modulates appetite and has shown potential for neuropathic pain management.

4. Delta-8 THC:

- Similar to Delta-9 THC but with milder psychoactive effects.

- Emerging research suggests analgesic and anti-inflammatory properties.

Current Research on Cannabis and Pain Relief

The scientific community has conducted extensive research on the efficacy of cannabis for pain management, encompassing clinical trials, systematic reviews, and preclinical studies.

1. Clinical Evidence

1. Neuropathic Pain:

A 2018 systematic review found that cannabis-based medicines significantly reduced neuropathic pain in patients with conditions such as multiple sclerosis and post-chemotherapy neuropathy.

2. Cancer Pain:

Studies reveal that cannabis reduces pain intensity in cancer patients, often allowing for reduced opioid use.

3. Arthritis and Inflammatory Pain:

Research demonstrates that CBD-rich cannabis oils and topicals alleviate joint pain and improve mobility in patients with rheumatoid arthritis and osteoarthritis.

2. Comparative Studies with Conventional Treatments

- Cannabis vs. Opioids:

Cannabis for Chronic Pain: A Nutritionist's Guide to Relief

- Cannabis offers comparable pain relief for some conditions with a lower risk of addiction and fewer side effects.
- Patients using cannabis report decreased reliance on opioids, highlighting its potential role in addressing the opioid epidemic.

- Cannabis vs. NSAIDs:
 - Particularly beneficial for long-term use, cannabis avoids the gastrointestinal and cardiovascular side effects associated with NSAIDs.

3. Preclinical Studies

- Animal models consistently demonstrate cannabis's efficacy in reducing both inflammatory and neuropathic pain.
- Studies on cannabinoids like CBG and THCV suggest expanding therapeutic possibilities beyond THC and CBD.

4. Limitations and Challenges in Research

1. Regulatory Barriers:
   - Legal restrictions on cannabis research hinder large-scale clinical trials.

2. Heterogeneity in Study Designs:
   - Variability in cannabis strains, dosages, and delivery methods complicates data interpretation.

3. Placebo Effect:
   - High placebo responses in pain studies highlight the need for rigorous trial designs.

Practical Applications of Cannabis for Pain Relief

1. Delivery Methods

- **Inhalation**: Provides rapid pain relief but with a shorter duration.
- **Oral Consumption:** Longer-lasting effects, ideal for chronic conditions.
- **Topicals**: Localized relief without systemic effects, useful for arthritis and muscle pain.
- **Transdermal Patches**: Consistent delivery for sustained pain relief.

2. Dosing Strategies

- **Start Low, Go Slow**: Gradual titration minimizes side effects and determines the optimal therapeutic dose.

- **Microdosing**: Small doses throughout the day can maintain steady pain relief without impairing function.

3. Combining Cannabinoids

- **Entourage Effect**: The synergistic interaction of cannabinoids, terpenes, and flavonoids enhances therapeutic efficacy.
- Products combining THC and CBD in varying ratios cater to specific pain profiles.

Cannabis's complex interaction with the ECS and other biological systems positions it as a versatile tool for pain management. THC, CBD, and other cannabinoids offer targeted relief for diverse pain conditions, supported by a growing body of research. However, challenges such as regulatory constraints and dosing variability underscore the need for continued investigation and patient education.

By integrating cannabis with evidence-based practices, healthcare providers can harness its full potential to improve patient outcomes.

Subsequent chapters will explore the nutritional implications of cannabis use and its integration into holistic pain management plans.

1.3: Nutrition and Chronic Pain: The Basics

Chronic pain affects millions worldwide, influencing quality of life and overall health. While pharmacological and alternative therapies are widely used for pain management, the role of nutrition is increasingly recognized as a cornerstone of holistic treatment. This chapter explores the impact of nutrition on chronic pain, identifies key nutrients and dietary patterns beneficial for pain management, and introduces the concept of "food as medicine." By integrating dietary strategies with other interventions, individuals can address pain at its roots and enhance their well-being.

Cannabis for Chronic Pain: A Nutritionist's Guide to Relief

The Impact of Nutrition on Chronic Pain

Nutrition directly influences the body's inflammatory processes, gut microbiome, and cellular health, all of which are critical in the context of chronic pain.

1. The Inflammatory Connection

1. Pro-Inflammatory vs. Anti-Inflammatory Diets:
   - Chronic pain is often linked to low-grade inflammation. Diets high in processed foods, refined sugars, and unhealthy fats can exacerbate this inflammation.
   - Conversely, diets rich in whole foods, healthy fats, and phytonutrients reduce inflammatory markers like C-reactive protein (CRP) and cytokines.

Cannabis for Chronic Pain: A Nutritionist's Guide to Relief

2. The Role of Omega-6 and Omega-3 Fatty Acids:

- Omega-6 Fatty Acids: Found in processed oils, excessive intake can promote inflammation.
- Omega-3 Fatty Acids: Found in fatty fish, flaxseeds, and walnuts, these fats counteract inflammation and alleviate pain, particularly in conditions like rheumatoid arthritis.

2. Gut Health and Pain Modulation

1. Gut Microbiome's Influence on Pain:

- Dysbiosis (an imbalance in gut bacteria) contributes to systemic inflammation, amplifying chronic pain.
- A healthy gut microbiome supports the production of short-chain fatty acids (SCFAs), which have anti-inflammatory effects.

2. Impact of Diet on Gut Health:

- High-fiber foods like vegetables, fruits, and whole grains nourish beneficial gut bacteria.
- Processed foods and antibiotics can disrupt the gut microbiome, worsening pain-related inflammation.

3. Blood Sugar Regulation and Pain

1. Hyperglycemia and Inflammation:
- Chronically high blood sugar levels from a diet high in refined carbs can increase oxidative stress and inflammation, intensifying pain.
- Balanced blood sugar through a low-glycemic diet helps mitigate these effects.

2. Role in Neuropathy:
- Conditions like diabetic neuropathy highlight the direct connection between poor glycemic control and nerve pain.

Cannabis for Chronic Pain: A Nutritionist's Guide to Relief

Key Nutrients and Dietary Patterns for Pain Management

Scientific evidence supports the inclusion of specific nutrients and dietary patterns to reduce chronic pain and improve overall health.

1. Anti-Inflammatory Nutrients

1. Omega-3 Fatty Acids:
   - **Sources**: Fatty fish (salmon, mackerel), chia seeds, walnuts.
   - **Benefits**: Reduce cytokine production, alleviate joint pain, and improve mobility in arthritis patients.

2. Vitamin D:
   - **Sources**: Sun exposure, fortified dairy, fatty fish, and mushrooms.

- **Benefits**: Plays a role in immune modulation and has been shown to reduce musculoskeletal pain.

3. **Magnesium:**
   - **Sources**: Dark leafy greens, nuts, seeds, and whole grains.
   - **Benefits**: Essential for nerve function, magnesium deficiency has been linked to migraines and fibromyalgia.

4. **Curcumin (from Turmeric):**
   - **Sources**: Turmeric root or supplements.
   - **Benefits**: Potent anti-inflammatory properties proven effective for osteoarthritis and inflammatory bowel disease.

5. **Polyphenols:**
   - **Sources**: Berries, green tea, dark chocolate, and olive oil.

- **Benefits**: Reduce oxidative stress and inflammation, contributing to pain relief in conditions like fibromyalgia.

2. Pain-Reducing Dietary Patterns

1. Mediterranean Diet:
  - **Features**: High in fruits, vegetables, whole grains, lean proteins, and healthy fats.
  - **Evidence**: Studies demonstrate its effectiveness in reducing inflammatory markers and chronic pain.

2. Plant-Based Diets:
  - **Features**: Focus on whole plant foods, minimal animal products.
  - **Evidence**: Shown to lower inflammation and improve pain in conditions like rheumatoid arthritis.

3. Low FODMAP Diet:

- **Features**: Reduces fermentable oligosaccharides, disaccharides, monosaccharides, and polyols.
  - **Application**: Effective for managing pain associated with irritable bowel syndrome (IBS).

4. **Ketogenic Diet**:
  - **Features**: High-fat, low-carb regimen.
  - **Evidence**: Reduces pain and inflammation in neuropathic conditions by promoting ketone production.

Introduction to the Concept of "Food as Medicine"

The concept of "food as medicine" emphasizes the proactive role of nutrition in preventing and managing chronic conditions, including pain.

Cannabis for Chronic Pain: A Nutritionist's Guide to Relief

1. Historical Context

1. Hippocrates' Philosophy: "Let food be thy medicine and medicine be thy food" underscores the ancient understanding of nutrition's role in health.
2. Traditional Practices: Ayurvedic and Traditional Chinese Medicine systems have long used specific foods and herbs to alleviate pain and inflammation.

2. Modern Applications

1. Functional Foods:
   - Foods like turmeric, ginger, and garlic are incorporated into diets for their specific anti-inflammatory and pain-relieving properties.

- Fortified and enriched foods provide nutrients like omega-3s and vitamin D for targeted relief.

2. Nutraceuticals:
   - Supplements like curcumin, glucosamine, and fish oil bridge the gap between diet and pharmacology.

3. Personalized Nutrition:
   - Advances in nutrigenomics allow for dietary recommendations tailored to an individual's genetic makeup, optimizing pain management.

Practical Applications for Chronic Pain Management

Cannabis for Chronic Pain: A Nutritionist's Guide to Relief

1. Creating a Pain-Relief Diet Plan

1. Assessment:
   - Analyze dietary patterns to identify deficiencies and pro-inflammatory foods.

2. Inclusion of Key Nutrients:
   - Prioritize omega-3s, magnesium, and polyphenol-rich foods.

3. Meal Planning:
   - Incorporate anti-inflammatory foods into every meal.
   - Example: A breakfast of chia seed pudding with berries, a lunch of quinoa salad with leafy greens and olive oil, and a dinner featuring salmon with roasted vegetables.

2. Lifestyle Integration

1. Mindful Eating:

Cannabis for Chronic Pain: A Nutritionist's Guide to Relief

- Slow, mindful eating improves digestion and nutrient absorption, reducing gut-related inflammation.

2. Hydration:
   - Adequate water intake supports cellular function and helps flush inflammatory toxins.

3. Stress Reduction:
   - Chronic stress exacerbates pain; practices like yoga and meditation can complement dietary changes.

Current Research and Future Directions

1. Evidence from Clinical Studies

Cannabis for Chronic Pain: A Nutritionist's Guide to Relief

1. Dietary Interventions:

- Randomized trials show significant pain reduction with diets like the Mediterranean or plant-based plans.

2. Nutritional Supplements:

- Meta-analyses reveal consistent benefits of omega-3 and curcumin supplements in managing arthritis pain.

2. Emerging Areas of Study

1. Gut-Brain Axis:

- Exploring how gut microbiota manipulation through diet influences pain perception.

2. Epigenetics:

- Understanding how nutrition modifies gene expression related to inflammation and pain pathways.

Cannabis for Chronic Pain: A Nutritionist's Guide to Relief

Nutrition is a powerful, underutilized tool in chronic pain management. By addressing inflammation, supporting gut health, and providing essential nutrients, dietary interventions offer a complementary approach to traditional therapies. The integration of "food as medicine" into pain management not only reduces discomfort but also empowers individuals to take control of their health. Subsequent chapters will explore the interplay between cannabis and nutrition, providing a holistic framework for managing chronic pain effectively.

Part 2: Cannabis and Nutrition for Chronic Pain Management

2.1: Cannabis and Omega-3 Fatty Acids: A Powerful Pain-Relieving Combination

The management of chronic pain is multifaceted, requiring interventions that address inflammation, neurochemical imbalances, and overall health. Omega-3 fatty acids, known for their anti-inflammatory and neuroprotective properties, are an essential dietary component for pain relief. Recent research suggests a synergistic relationship between omega-3 fatty acids and cannabis, enhancing their pain-relieving effects through shared mechanisms in the endocannabinoid system. This chapter delves into the science behind omega-3 fatty acids in pain management, the interactions between cannabis and omega-3s, and how these two interventions work together to improve chronic pain outcomes.

Cannabis for Chronic Pain: A Nutritionist's Guide to Relief

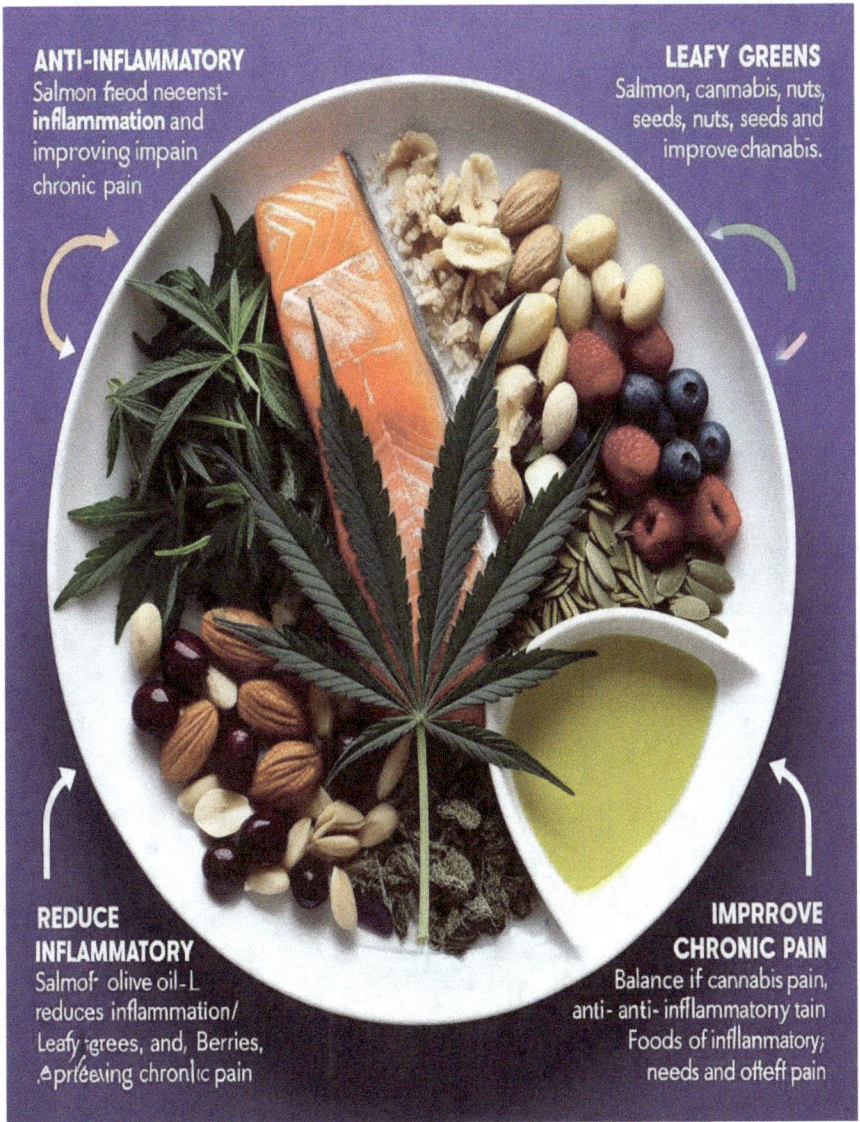

Nutritional Synergy with Cannabis

The Role of Omega-3 Fatty Acids in Pain Management

1. Understanding Omega-3 Fatty Acids

1. Types of Omega-3s:
   - **Alpha-Linolenic Acid (ALA):** Found in flaxseeds, chia seeds, and walnuts; a precursor to other omega-3s.
   - **Eicosapentaenoic Acid (EPA):** Found in fatty fish; directly involved in reducing inflammation.
   - **Docosahexaenoic Acid (DHA):** Found in fatty fish; critical for brain health and reducing neuroinflammation.

2. Biological Roles:
   - **Anti-Inflammatory Effects**: Omega-3s inhibit the production of pro-inflammatory cytokines and promote the synthesis of

resolvins and protectins, compounds that resolve inflammation.

- **Neurological Benefits**: DHA supports neuronal health, while EPA reduces neuroinflammation linked to pain perception.

- **Cellular Function**: Omega-3s maintain cell membrane fluidity, supporting the function of receptor systems, including the endocannabinoid system.

2. Mechanisms of Pain Relief

1. Reduction of Pro-Inflammatory Mediators:
   - Omega-3s suppress the production of prostaglandins and leukotrienes, reducing inflammation-related pain.

2. Modulation of Immune Responses:
   - By balancing the activity of immune cells, omega-3s decrease autoimmune responses that

exacerbate pain conditions like rheumatoid arthritis.

3. Impact on Neuropathic Pain:
   - Omega-3s repair damaged nerves and reduce oxidative stress, offering relief in conditions like diabetic neuropathy and fibromyalgia.

3. Clinical Evidence

1. Arthritis and Joint Pain:
   - Studies show that omega-3 supplementation significantly reduces joint pain, stiffness, and swelling in arthritis patients.

2. Neuropathic Pain:
   - Research demonstrates that omega-3s improve nerve function and reduce pain intensity in neuropathic conditions.

3. Headaches and Migraines:

Cannabis for Chronic Pain: A Nutritionist's Guide to Relief

- Omega-3s lower the frequency and severity of migraines, likely due to their anti-inflammatory and vasodilatory effects.

Cannabis and Omega-3 Fatty Acids: Mechanistic Interactions

1. The Endocannabinoid System and Omega-3s

1. Endocannabinoid Precursors:
   - Omega-3s are precursors to endocannabinoids like anandamide (AEA) and 2-arachidonoylglycerol (2-AG). These lipid-based neurotransmitters play a crucial role in pain modulation.

2. Enhancing Receptor Function:

Cannabis for Chronic Pain: A Nutritionist's Guide to Relief

   - Omega-3s improve the binding affinity of cannabinoids to CB1 and CB2 receptors, amplifying the effects of both endocannabinoids and phytocannabinoids.

3. Regulation of Enzymatic Activity:
   - Omega-3s inhibit enzymes like fatty acid amide hydrolase (FAAH) that degrade endocannabinoids, prolonging their pain-relieving effects.

2. Cannabis Synergy with Omega-3s

1. THC and Omega-3s:
   - **Mechanism**: THC activates CB1 receptors in the brain and central nervous system, reducing pain perception. Omega-3s enhance this activation by maintaining receptor health.
   - **Effect**: Improved pain relief with fewer side effects like tolerance or dependency.

2. CBD and Omega-3s:

- **Mechanism**: CBD interacts with non-cannabinoid receptors and modulates inflammatory pathways. Omega-3s support these actions by reducing baseline inflammation.
- **Effect**: Enhanced anti-inflammatory and neuroprotective benefits.

3. Combination Therapy Benefits:

- Reduced reliance on high doses of THC or CBD, minimizing psychoactive side effects and cost.

Current Research on Cannabis and Omega-3s in Pain Relief

Cannabis for Chronic Pain: A Nutritionist's Guide to Relief

1. Preclinical Studies

1. Inflammatory Pain Models:
  - Animal studies show that omega-3 supplementation enhances the analgesic effects of THC and CBD in reducing inflammatory pain.

2. Neuropathic Pain Models:
  - Combining omega-3s with cannabinoids improves nerve regeneration and reduces hyperalgesia in rodent models of neuropathy.

2. Clinical Studies

1. Arthritis Trials:
  - Preliminary trials indicate that patients using both cannabis and omega-3 supplements report greater reductions in joint pain and improved mobility compared to either intervention alone.

2. Cancer Pain Management:

 - Patients with chemotherapy-induced neuropathy experience significant pain relief when combining cannabinoids with omega-3s, highlighting the synergy between the two.

3. Migraine Relief:

 - A combination of omega-3s and cannabis reduces the frequency and intensity of migraines, outperforming monotherapies.

3. Ongoing Research Areas

1. Dosing Strategies:

 - Studies aim to determine optimal ratios of omega-3s to cannabinoids for various pain conditions.

2. Long-Term Safety:

Cannabis for Chronic Pain: A Nutritionist's Guide to Relief

- Research focuses on the safety of chronic combined use, particularly concerning cardiovascular and neurological health.

Practical Applications: Integrating Cannabis and Omega-3s for Pain Relief

1. Dietary Recommendations

1. Sources of Omega-3s:
 - **Natural Foods:** Fatty fish, flaxseeds, chia seeds, walnuts.
 - **Supplements**: High-quality fish oil or algae-based omega-3 supplements for those with dietary restrictions.

2. Balancing Omega-6 to Omega-3 Ratio:

- Reduce intake of processed seed oils high in omega-6 fatty acids.

2. Cannabis Administration

1. Forms:
- THC and CBD oils, capsules, edibles, or topical formulations can be paired with omega-3-rich meals.

2. Dosing:
- Start with low doses of cannabinoids and gradually increase while maintaining consistent omega-3 intake.

3. Combined Therapy Protocol

1. Step 1: Dietary Assessment
- Evaluate omega-3 intake and supplement if necessary.

2. **Step 2:** Introduce Cannabis
   - Use CBD-rich or balanced THC:CBD products for anti-inflammatory benefits.

3. **Step 3:** Monitor Outcomes
   - Track pain levels, side effects, and overall well-being to adjust the therapy plan.

The combination of cannabis and omega-3 fatty acids represents a promising strategy for managing chronic pain. Through complementary mechanisms, these interventions address inflammation, neuronal health, and pain modulation at multiple levels. As research evolves, integrating cannabis and omega-3s into personalized treatment plans offers a path toward improved quality of life for those suffering from chronic pain. The next chapter will explore the broader role of nutrition in optimizing cannabis-based therapies, expanding on this powerful synergy.

2.2: The Impact of Cannabis on Gut Health and Chronic Pain

The relationship between gut health and chronic pain is deeply rooted in the bidirectional communication of the gut-brain axis. This complex system connects the central nervous system (CNS) with the gastrointestinal (GI) tract, significantly influencing pain perception and overall health. Cannabis, with its impact on both the endocannabinoid system (ECS) and gut physiology, offers promising therapeutic potential for managing gut-related chronic pain. This chapter explores the interplay between the gut-brain axis, cannabis, and nutrition, focusing on strategies to optimize both gut health and the efficacy of cannabis-based interventions.

The Gut-Brain Axis and Its Role in Chronic Pain

1. Anatomy and Function of the Gut-Brain Axis

1. Bidirectional Communication:
   - The gut-brain axis connects the CNS and enteric nervous system (ENS) through neural, hormonal, and immune pathways.
   - Key players include the vagus nerve, gut microbiota, and neurotransmitters like serotonin and gamma-aminobutyric acid (GABA).

2. Gut Microbiota:
   - Comprising trillions of microorganisms, the gut microbiota plays a critical role in modulating inflammation, immunity, and pain signaling.

Cannabis for Chronic Pain: A Nutritionist's Guide to Relief

- Dysbiosis (microbial imbalance) is linked to conditions like irritable bowel syndrome (IBS), fibromyalgia, and chronic inflammatory states.

3. Neurotransmitters and Pain Perception:

- The gut produces over 90% of the body's serotonin, a neurotransmitter involved in mood and pain regulation.
- Alterations in gut neurotransmitter levels can directly impact chronic pain conditions.

2. Gut-Related Pain Pathways

1. Visceral Pain:

- Originates from internal organs, often associated with conditions like IBS and inflammatory bowel disease (IBD).

2. Peripheral and Central Sensitization:

- Persistent gut inflammation can lead to heightened sensitivity in pain pathways, contributing to chronic pain syndromes.

3. Role of Immune Activation:
   - Chronic pain is exacerbated by the release of pro-inflammatory cytokines and immune mediators from the gut.

3. Clinical Evidence of Gut-Brain Axis in Chronic Pain

1. IBS and Chronic Pain:
   - Studies show a strong correlation between gut health and symptom severity in IBS and other functional GI disorders.

2. Fibromyalgia and Gut Dysbiosis:
   - Emerging research suggests that patients with fibromyalgia often exhibit altered gut microbiota, linking gut health to widespread pain.

Cannabis for Chronic Pain: A Nutritionist's Guide to Relief

How Cannabis Affects Gut Health and Chronic Pain

1. The Endocannabinoid System in the Gut

1. CB1 and CB2 Receptors:
   - CB1 receptors are found in the ENS and regulate motility, secretion, and visceral sensitivity.
   - CB2 receptors are involved in immune modulation and reducing gut inflammation.

2. Endocannabinoids:
   - Anandamide (AEA) and 2-arachidonoylglycerol (2-AG) play key roles in maintaining gut homeostasis and modulating pain signals.

3. Gut Microbiota Interaction:
   - ECS signaling is influenced by the gut microbiota, creating a feedback loop that impacts inflammation and pain perception.

Cannabis for Chronic Pain: A Nutritionist's Guide to Relief

2. Cannabis and Inflammation in the Gut

1. Anti-Inflammatory Properties:
   - THC and CBD reduce pro-inflammatory cytokine production and inhibit immune cell infiltration in the gut lining.

2. Modulation of Gut Barrier Function:
   - Cannabis compounds help maintain the integrity of the intestinal barrier, preventing "leaky gut" and systemic inflammation.

3. Role in Autoimmune Conditions:
   - Cannabis has shown promise in reducing symptoms of Crohn's disease, ulcerative colitis, and other autoimmune-related gut disorders.

3. Cannabis and Gut Motility

1. THC and Gastrointestinal Transit:

- THC slows gut motility, offering relief for diarrhea-predominant conditions.

2. **CBD and Smooth Muscle Function**:
 - CBD relaxes smooth muscle contractions, reducing spasms and discomfort in GI disorders.

4. Clinical Evidence: Cannabis for Gut-Related Chronic Pain

1. IBS:
 - Studies highlight significant symptom relief in IBS patients using cannabis, particularly for abdominal pain and bloating.

2. IBD:
 - Cannabis use is associated with reduced inflammation, improved quality of life, and decreased reliance on corticosteroids in IBD patients.

Cannabis for Chronic Pain: A Nutritionist's Guide to Relief

3. Chronic Pain Syndromes:

 - Patients with fibromyalgia and overlapping GI symptoms report improved pain and gut health with cannabinoid therapies.

Nutritional Strategies for Promoting Gut Health and Cannabis Efficacy

1. The Role of Diet in Gut Health

1. Prebiotics:

 - Foods rich in prebiotics (e.g., garlic, onions, asparagus) fuel beneficial gut bacteria, supporting ECS balance.

2. Probiotics:

 - Fermented foods (e.g., yogurt, sauerkraut, kimchi) introduce beneficial bacteria, improving gut microbiota diversity and resilience.

3. Anti-Inflammatory Foods:
   - Include omega-3 fatty acids, leafy greens, and spices like turmeric to reduce systemic and gut inflammation.

4. Fiber-Rich Diet:
   - Soluble and insoluble fibers support gut motility and microbiota diversity, improving ECS function.

2. Optimizing Cannabis Efficacy Through Nutrition

1. Fat-Soluble Cannabinoids:
   - Consuming cannabis with healthy fats (e.g., avocados, nuts, olive oil) enhances absorption of THC and CBD.

2. Omega-3 Fatty Acids:

Cannabis for Chronic Pain: A Nutritionist's Guide to Relief

- As discussed in the previous chapter, omega-3s optimize ECS functionality, enhancing cannabis efficacy.

3. Micronutrients:

- Magnesium, zinc, and vitamin D support ECS health and pain relief.

3. Diet Plans for Gut and Pain Management

1. Elimination Diets:

- Identify and remove trigger foods (e.g., gluten, dairy) that exacerbate gut inflammation and chronic pain.

2. Mediterranean Diet:

- Emphasizes anti-inflammatory foods, healthy fats, and whole grains, complementing cannabis-based therapies.

3. Low-FODMAP Diet:

- Reduces fermentable carbohydrates, alleviating symptoms of IBS and related pain syndromes.

Practical Applications and Case Studies

1. Integrating Cannabis and Gut-Healthy Nutrition

- Develop personalized plans combining cannabis, dietary adjustments, and probiotics.
- Monitor patient outcomes through symptom tracking and regular assessments.

2. Case Study: IBS and Cannabis

- **Background**: 38-year-old female with IBS-D and chronic abdominal pain.

Cannabis for Chronic Pain: A Nutritionist's Guide to Relief

- **Intervention**: High-CBD cannabis oil with a low-FODMAP diet and prebiotic supplementation.
- **Outcome**: Significant reduction in pain and improved bowel regularity within three months.

3. Case Study: Fibromyalgia with Gut Dysbiosis

- **Background**: 52-year-old male with fibromyalgia and bloating.
- **Intervention**: Balanced THC:CBD tincture alongside a Mediterranean diet and probiotics.
- **Outcome**: Decreased pain severity and reduced gut discomfort within six weeks.

The gut-brain axis plays a pivotal role in chronic pain, making gut health a critical component of pain management strategies. Cannabis offers unique benefits for modulating gut physiology and alleviating pain, while dietary interventions optimize its efficacy. Together, cannabis and nutrition provide a comprehensive, integrative approach to chronic pain relief, addressing the underlying mechanisms and improving patient outcomes. In the next chapter, we will explore the role of cannabis and antioxidants in managing inflammation and oxidative stress, further advancing our understanding of cannabis-based nutritional therapies.

2.3: Cannabis, Magnesium, and Muscle Relaxation: A Trio for Pain Relief

Chronic pain, especially pain linked with muscle spasms, is a common challenge faced by many individuals. In the quest for effective pain relief, the combination of cannabis and magnesium offers a unique approach to managing pain by targeting muscle relaxation and overall pain mitigation. Both substances have demonstrated significant benefits for individuals with muscle-related chronic pain, such as fibromyalgia, arthritis, and other musculoskeletal disorders.

This chapter explores the synergistic relationship between cannabis and magnesium in managing muscle-related pain. We will examine the roles of each compound individually in muscle relaxation and pain

Cannabis for Chronic Pain: A Nutritionist's Guide to Relief

management, how they interact to amplify pain relief, and discuss strategies for optimizing their effectiveness through diet and supplementation.

Cannabis for Chronic Pain: A Nutritionist's Guide to Relief

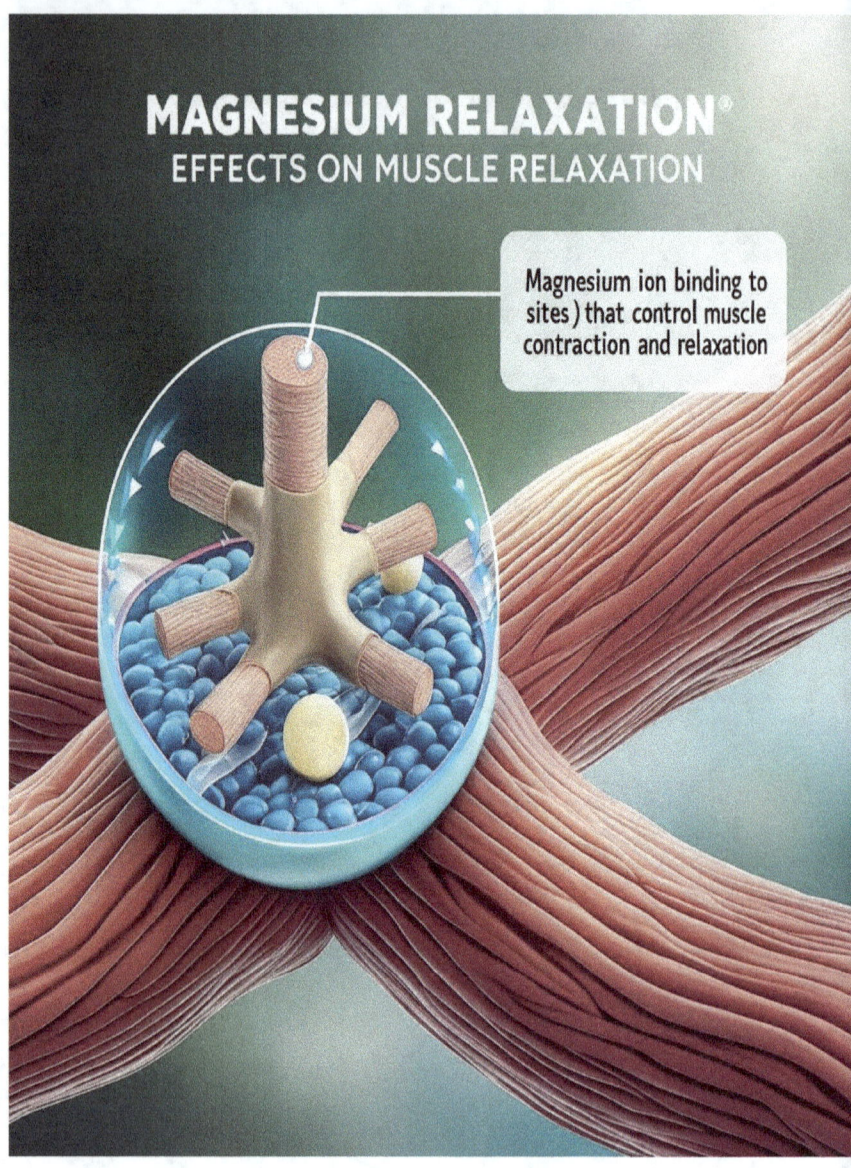

Magnesium's Role in Muscle Relaxation

Cannabis for Chronic Pain: A Nutritionist's Guide to Relief

1. The Role of Magnesium in Muscle Relaxation and Pain Management

Magnesium is a vital mineral that plays numerous roles in maintaining bodily function, including its essential role in muscle function. It is involved in over 300 enzymatic processes within the body, many of which are crucial for muscle relaxation and the management of pain.

1.1. Magnesium and Muscle Function

Magnesium plays a key role in muscle contraction and relaxation. Muscle fibers depend on magnesium to regulate the flow of calcium ions, which are necessary for muscle contraction. When magnesium levels are deficient, muscles can become hyper-excitable, leading to muscle spasms, cramps, and tightness. This condition is commonly observed in individuals experiencing chronic pain conditions like fibromyalgia or tension-type headaches.

- **Calcium and Magnesium Balance**: Calcium triggers muscle contraction, while magnesium is necessary for muscle relaxation. A deficiency in magnesium disrupts this balance, leading to prolonged muscle contractions (spasms) and increased pain sensitivity.

- **Muscle Relaxation**: Magnesium acts as a natural muscle relaxant by helping to neutralize excess calcium in muscle cells, which allows muscles to relax more fully.

1.2. Magnesium's Role in Pain Modulation

Magnesium also influences the body's ability to process pain signals. It does so by regulating the NMDA (N-Methyl-D-Aspartate) receptor, which plays a significant role in pain perception. An overactive NMDA receptor is linked to the heightened pain sensitivity observed in many chronic pain conditions. Magnesium acts as a natural blocker of NMDA receptors, thus reducing the pain sensation.

- **Pain Pathways**: Magnesium has been shown to modulate several pain pathways, reducing the body's sensitivity to pain by controlling neurotransmitter release and diminishing central sensitization (the process by which the central nervous system becomes hypersensitive to pain).

- **Anti-Inflammatory Properties**: Magnesium also exerts anti-inflammatory effects, which are vital in reducing the inflammation that often accompanies muscle spasms and pain.

1.3. Research Supporting Magnesium's Role in Pain Relief

Numerous studies have explored magnesium's role in muscle relaxation and chronic pain management. For example:

- **Fibromyalgia**: In a 2012 study published in the **Journal of Rheumatology**, researchers found that magnesium supplementation helped reduce pain, fatigue, and anxiety in patients with fibromyalgia, a condition often characterized by widespread muscle pain.
- **Migraine Relief**: Magnesium is well known for its ability to reduce the frequency and severity of migraines, a type of chronic pain linked to muscle tension in the neck and scalp.
- **General Pain Relief**: A review of several clinical studies concluded that magnesium supplementation is associated with significant reductions in pain intensity, especially in patients with chronic pain conditions like arthritis and lower back pain.

2. How Cannabis and Magnesium Interact to Enhance Pain Relief

Cannabis, particularly its cannabinoids THC (tetrahydrocannabinol) and CBD (cannabidiol), has shown promise in relieving chronic pain. The combination of cannabis with magnesium could offer a more potent solution to managing muscle-related pain. Understanding how cannabis and magnesium work together to enhance muscle relaxation and pain relief is key to maximizing their therapeutic potential.

2.1. Cannabis and the Endocannabinoid System (ECS)

Cannabinoids, such as THC and CBD, interact with the body's endocannabinoid system (ECS), a complex signaling system that helps regulate various physiological processes, including pain, inflammation, and muscle relaxation. The ECS consists of cannabinoid receptors (CB1 and CB2), endocannabinoids (naturally occurring compounds in the body), and enzymes that help break down these compounds.

- **CB1 and CB2 Receptors**: THC, the psychoactive cannabinoid, binds primarily to CB1 receptors located in the brain and central nervous system, helping to modulate pain perception. CBD, on the other hand, interacts with both CB1 and CB2 receptors, though its effects are less direct and more modulatory. By activating or inhibiting these receptors, cannabinoids can influence pain pathways.
- **Pain Modulation**: Cannabis works by interacting with the ECS to modulate pain perception, reduce inflammation, and enhance muscle relaxation. THC is particularly effective at reducing pain intensity, while CBD may contribute to pain relief by mitigating the stress response and reducing inflammation.

2.2. The Synergy Between Magnesium and Cannabis

When used together, cannabis and magnesium have a complementary effect on muscle relaxation and pain management. The combined action of cannabinoids and magnesium provides an enhanced therapeutic effect due to their shared mechanisms of action and their ability to target multiple pain pathways.

- **Muscle Relaxation**: Both magnesium and cannabis work to promote muscle relaxation, albeit through different mechanisms. Magnesium relaxes muscles by influencing calcium channels and the NMDA receptors, while cannabis acts on the ECS to reduce pain and inflammation.
- **Pain Relief**: Magnesium's ability to block NMDA receptors can synergize with cannabis's

influence on the ECS, providing a dual approach to reducing pain. Additionally, cannabis's anti-inflammatory properties may enhance magnesium's ability to reduce muscle inflammation and pain.

2.3. Research on Cannabis and Magnesium Interaction

While the research on the direct interaction between cannabis and magnesium is still developing, studies have shown promising results:

- **Combination Effects**: Research suggests that combining cannabinoids with other natural compounds like magnesium can produce an enhanced effect on pain relief and muscle relaxation. For instance, a study published in **Frontiers in Pharmacology** highlighted how CBD enhanced the effectiveness of magnesium in reducing muscle spasticity.

- **Cannabis for Muscle Spasms**: Cannabis has been widely studied for its ability to reduce muscle spasms and chronic pain in conditions like multiple sclerosis (MS). Magnesium's muscle-relaxing properties may work synergistically with cannabis to further alleviate spasticity and muscle-related pain in MS patients.

3. Nutritional Strategies for Optimizing Magnesium Levels and Cannabis Efficacy

To optimize the effectiveness of both magnesium and cannabis in managing chronic pain, it is essential to ensure that magnesium levels are maintained at optimal levels and that cannabis is used appropriately. The following strategies can help enhance the efficacy of these two compounds.

3.1. Dietary Sources of Magnesium

Incorporating magnesium-rich foods into the diet is the first step toward improving magnesium levels. Magnesium can be found in a variety of whole foods, including:

- **Leafy Green Vegetables**: Spinach, kale, and Swiss chard are excellent sources of magnesium.
- **Nuts and Seeds**: Almonds, cashews, pumpkin seeds, and sunflower seeds are magnesium-rich snacks.
- **Whole Grains**: Brown rice, quinoa, and oats provide significant amounts of magnesium.
- **Legumes**: Lentils, beans, and chickpeas are great plant-based sources of magnesium.

- **Fish**: Fatty fish such as salmon and mackerel contain both magnesium and anti-inflammatory omega-3 fatty acids.

3.2. Magnesium Supplementation

For individuals who are unable to obtain adequate magnesium from their diet, supplementation may be necessary. The recommended daily allowance (RDA) for magnesium varies based on age and gender, but generally, adult women need about 310-320 mg per day, and men require 400-420 mg per day. Magnesium supplements come in several forms, including:

- **Magnesium Citrate**: Highly bioavailable and commonly used for pain management.
- **Magnesium Glycinate**: Known for its calming effects and minimal laxative effect.
- **Magnesium Malate**: Often used for fibromyalgia and chronic fatigue syndrome.

3.3. Optimizing Cannabis Use for Pain Relief

To maximize the benefits of cannabis for pain relief, consider the following:

- **Choose the Right Cannabinoids:** THC is particularly effective for acute pain relief, while CBD is better suited for long-term pain management and inflammation reduction.
- **Proper Dosage**: Start with low doses of THC and CBD and gradually increase to find the optimal dosage. Overuse of THC may lead to psychoactive effects, which can be counterproductive in pain management.
- **Method of Consumption**: The method of cannabis consumption can affect its potency and onset of action. Smoking or vaporizing cannabis provides rapid relief, while edibles offer longer-lasting effects but take longer to kick in.

3.4. Combining Magnesium and Cannabis in Treatment Plans

Integrating magnesium-rich foods and supplements with cannabis use may significantly enhance pain relief. A balanced approach involves:

- **Dietary and Supplementation Support:** Ensure consistent intake of magnesium through food and, when necessary, supplements.
- **Cannabis Integration**: Use cannabis in a way that complements magnesium intake, such as using it for acute pain relief when magnesium supplementation supports long-term pain management.

Cannabis and magnesium form a potent duo in managing chronic pain, particularly for those suffering from muscle spasms and tension. While magnesium plays a crucial role in muscle relaxation and pain modulation,

Cannabis for Chronic Pain: A Nutritionist's Guide to Relief

cannabis enhances this effect through its interaction with the endocannabinoid system and its anti-inflammatory properties. By incorporating both substances into a comprehensive treatment plan, individuals with chronic pain can experience

Part 3: Putting it All Together – A Comprehensive Approach to Cannabis and Nutrition for Chronic Pain

3.1: Creating a Personalized Cannabis and Nutrition Plan for Chronic Pain

Chronic pain affects millions of people worldwide, and its management requires a multi-faceted approach that addresses the underlying causes and offers relief from the symptoms. While pharmacological treatments such as pain medications have long been the standard, many individuals seek alternative therapies that offer fewer side effects and promote overall wellness. Cannabis and nutrition are two such complementary approaches that can be effectively integrated into a holistic treatment plan for chronic pain management.

This chapter provides a comprehensive guide for creating a personalized cannabis and nutrition plan tailored to individual needs, health status, and chronic pain conditions. It explores how to assess individual health needs, set achievable goals, develop a treatment plan that integrates cannabis and nutritional strategies, and continually monitor and adjust the plan based on progress and feedback. With the increasing acceptance of cannabis in pain management, it is crucial for healthcare providers and individuals to develop personalized strategies that promote both short- and long-term relief.

Cannabis for Chronic Pain: A Nutritionist's Guide to Relief

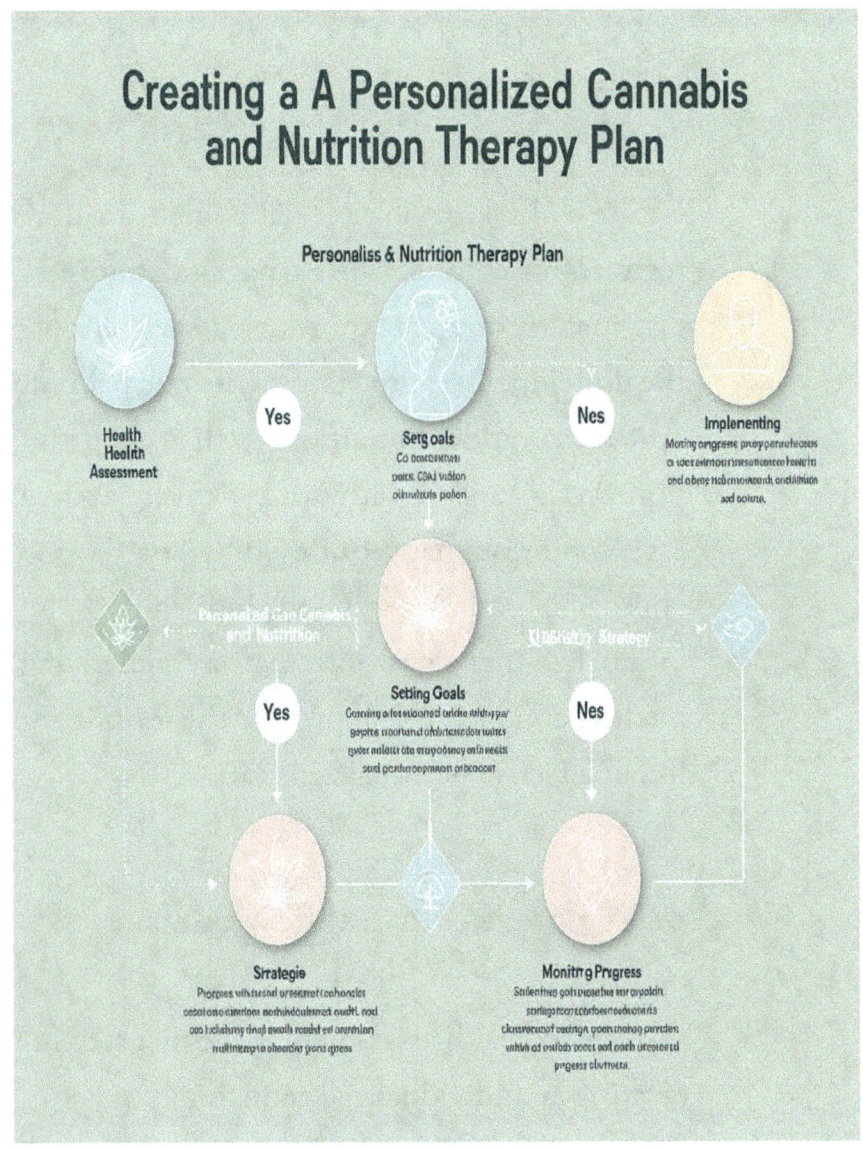

Personalized Cannabis and Nutrition Plan

Cannabis for Chronic Pain: A Nutritionist's Guide to Relief

1. Assessing Individual Needs and Health Status

Before embarking on a cannabis and nutrition regimen for chronic pain management, it is essential to conduct a thorough assessment of the individual's health status. Chronic pain can arise from various conditions such as arthritis, fibromyalgia, neuropathy, or back pain, and each condition may require a different approach. Understanding the individual's overall health, pain profile, and any underlying medical conditions will provide the foundation for an effective personalized plan.

1.1. Comprehensive Health Assessment

A detailed health assessment is the first step in creating an individualized cannabis and nutrition plan. This includes evaluating both physical and psychological factors that could influence pain and pain management strategies.

- **Pain History**: Documenting the type, intensity, and duration of pain is critical. Assess the pain's location, its frequency, triggers, and any previous treatments used.
- **Comorbidities**: Identify other medical conditions such as gastrointestinal issues, cardiovascular disease, kidney or liver function, or mental health concerns like anxiety or depression. These factors can influence the choice of cannabis strains, nutrients, and overall treatment plan.
- **Medications and Supplements**: Review current medications and supplements. Some drugs may interact with cannabis or affect nutrient absorption, while certain nutritional deficiencies might exacerbate chronic pain.
- **Lifestyle Factors**: Evaluate sleep patterns, physical activity levels, stress, diet, and any behaviors that may impact pain and overall

health. Chronic pain often leads to decreased physical activity and poor sleep, which can create a vicious cycle.

1.2. Pain Profile and Type of Pain

The nature of the pain—whether it is nociceptive (due to tissue injury), neuropathic (nerve damage), or inflammatory—can significantly influence the treatment approach. Different pain types respond to different forms of cannabis and nutritional interventions.

- **Nociceptive Pain**: This pain, caused by tissue damage or inflammation, may benefit from anti-inflammatory nutrients and cannabis strains with higher CBD content.
- **Neuropathic Pain**: Nerve-related pain, often described as burning or shooting, may require cannabis strains higher in THC and certain B-vitamins to address nerve regeneration.

- **Muscle Spasms and Spasticity**: Magnesium, together with cannabis, may be particularly effective in treating muscle spasms and tension. Magnesium is a critical mineral involved in muscle relaxation, and cannabis may help modulate pain signals and reduce inflammation.

1.3. Personal Preferences and Treatment Goals

Understanding a patient's preferences regarding the form of cannabis (e.g., oils, tinctures, edibles, or vaporizers) and the type of diet they follow (e.g., vegan, keto, low-carb) is important for creating a sustainable plan. Treatment goals should also be discussed and prioritized.

- **Goals of Treatment**: These may range from complete pain relief to simply improving mobility or reducing medication reliance. It is crucial to align the cannabis and nutrition plan with realistic, achievable outcomes.

- **Quality of Life Considerations**: Some individuals may prioritize quality of life improvements such as better sleep, reduced anxiety, or enhanced mood, which can also be supported by the right combination of cannabis and nutrients.

2. Setting Goals and Developing a Treatment Plan

Once a comprehensive health assessment is complete, the next step is to set clear and measurable goals for pain management and develop a tailored treatment plan. The plan should combine appropriate cannabis strains, dosages, and delivery methods with nutritional strategies aimed at supporting the body's healing and pain reduction processes.

2.1. Defining Treatment Goals

Treatment goals must be specific, measurable, and attainable. Working with the individual, healthcare providers can outline desired outcomes, such as:

- **Pain Reduction**: A reduction in pain intensity and frequency, measurable through self-reports or pain scales.
- **Improved Mobility**: Achieving greater physical function or movement, particularly in those with joint pain or muscle spasms.
- **Reduced Inflammation**: Reducing inflammation markers through dietary changes or anti-inflammatory cannabis compounds like CBD.

- **Improved Sleep**: Addressing the common issue of sleep disturbances in chronic pain patients, as proper sleep is crucial for pain management.

- **Reduced Dependence on Opioids or Other Medications**: Many individuals with chronic pain are looking to reduce their use of prescription painkillers. A successful cannabis and nutrition plan may help taper these medications safely.

2.2. Developing a Personalized Cannabis Plan

The next step is to create a cannabis plan that aligns with the individual's pain profile and treatment goals. The cannabis plan should consider both the choice of cannabis strains and the delivery method, as these factors will influence both the onset and duration of pain relief.

Cannabis for Chronic Pain: A Nutritionist's Guide to Relief

- **Cannabis Strains**: Different strains of cannabis offer varied effects. For example:

  - **Indica Strains**: Known for their relaxing and sedative properties, these strains may be ideal for individuals dealing with insomnia or muscle spasms.

  - **Sativa Strains**: Often uplifting and energizing, sativa strains can be useful for daytime pain management, helping to improve mood and focus.

  - **Hybrid Strains**: A combination of indica and sativa, hybrids may offer balanced effects, addressing both pain and mood.

- **THC vs. CBD**: THC is known for its pain-relieving properties but may cause psychoactive effects, which some patients may find undesirable. CBD, while non-psychoactive, has strong anti-inflammatory and pain-relieving effects and is often used for long-term management.

- **Dosage**: The proper dosage is highly individualized. Starting with a low dose and gradually increasing is crucial to avoid potential side effects and to find the optimal dosage for pain relief.

- **Delivery Methods**: Different methods of cannabis delivery offer distinct benefits:

  - **Inhalation (vaping/smoking):** Provides quick relief, making it ideal for acute pain management.

  - **Edibles**: Offer long-lasting effects, though they take longer to take effect. Ideal for sustained pain relief.

  - **Tinctures and Oils**: Provide flexibility in dosing and can be taken sublingually for rapid absorption.

2.3. Nutritional Strategies to Support Pain Relief

Nutrition plays a vital role in pain management. A diet rich in anti-inflammatory foods, essential vitamins, and minerals can support the body's healing processes and enhance the effectiveness of cannabis therapy.

- **Anti-Inflammatory Diet**: Incorporating foods like omega-3 fatty acids (found in fatty fish, flaxseeds, and walnuts), turmeric, ginger, and antioxidants can help reduce inflammation and complement the pain-relieving effects of cannabis.

- **Magnesium**: Ensuring adequate magnesium intake can help relax muscles and prevent spasms. Magnesium-rich foods (leafy greens, seeds, nuts, legumes) or supplements can help reduce muscle-related pain and improve overall muscle function.

- **Vitamin D and Calcium**: These nutrients are essential for bone health and may help with pain caused by musculoskeletal disorders like arthritis. Vitamin D can also influence the body's response to cannabinoids.

- **Amino Acids:** Amino acids, particularly glutamine and arginine, support the body's recovery from muscle strain and injuries, promoting healing and reducing pain.

2.4. Integrating Cannabis and Nutrition

To optimize the effects of both cannabis and nutrition, it is important to create a plan that combines both elements. This may include:

- **Pairing Anti-Inflammatory Foods with Cannabis**: For instance, taking CBD oil with an omega-3-rich meal can enhance its anti-inflammatory effects.
- **Timing Nutrition with Cannabis**: Consuming magnesium-rich foods or supplements before using cannabis may improve the muscle-relaxing effects and reduce the likelihood of cramps and spasms.

3. Monitoring Progress and Adjusting the Plan

A key component of any successful chronic pain treatment plan is ongoing monitoring and adaptation. Chronic pain is dynamic and can change in intensity, location, and nature, so it is crucial to track the individual's progress and adjust the cannabis and nutrition plan as needed.

3.1. Regular Check-ins and Pain Tracking

Regular follow-up appointments or check-ins are essential for assessing the effectiveness of the plan. Pain scales, mood assessments, and physical function tests can help measure progress. Patients should also be encouraged to track their symptoms and any side effects.

- **Pain Diary**: Encouraging individuals to keep a pain diary can help identify patterns, triggers, and effective interventions.
- **Symptom Tracking Apps**: There are numerous apps available that allow patients to track pain, sleep, mood, and medication use.

3.2. Adjusting Dosage and Delivery Methods

Based on feedback, the cannabis dosage or delivery method may need to be adjusted. For instance, if a particular strain is not providing adequate relief, switching to a different strain or adjusting the dosage might be necessary.

- **Gradual Titration**: Increasing the cannabis dose slowly and carefully ensures that the patient doesn't experience negative side effects like dizziness or anxiety.
- **Change in Delivery Method**: If an oral cannabis product isn't providing sufficient

relief, switching to a vape or tincture may offer faster onset and stronger effects.

3.3. Adjusting Nutritional Strategies

Nutritional plans may also need to be modified based on progress. For example, if the patient is experiencing digestive issues or weight gain, the nutrition plan can be adjusted to focus on gut health or reducing inflammatory foods. Regular assessments of nutrient levels (e.g., magnesium, vitamin D) through blood tests or symptom tracking can guide dietary adjustments.

3.4. Feedback Loop and Continuous Improvement

An effective cannabis and nutrition plan should be fluid, with the flexibility to make improvements based on ongoing feedback.

Cannabis for Chronic Pain: A Nutritionist's Guide to Relief

Collaboration with healthcare professionals, including a nutritionist, pain specialist, or cannabis expert, ensures that the plan remains aligned with the individual's needs.

Creating a personalized cannabis and nutrition plan for chronic pain requires a comprehensive approach that takes into account the individual's unique health status, treatment goals, and preferences. By assessing pain profiles, setting realistic goals, and integrating cannabis with targeted nutritional strategies, healthcare providers can offer effective, holistic relief for those suffering from chronic pain. Monitoring progress and adjusting the plan based on individual feedback ensures that the treatment continues to evolve, providing the best possible outcomes for long-term pain management.

3.2: Cannabis and Nutrition Interactions: What to Watch Out For

The therapeutic use of cannabis for chronic pain is increasingly recognized as a valuable option, often used alongside medications and nutritional interventions. However, integrating cannabis into a treatment plan requires a careful understanding of its potential interactions with medications and nutritional considerations. These interactions can affect efficacy, increase the risk of side effects, and alter the body's metabolic processes. By addressing these challenges through informed strategies, practitioners and patients can maximize the benefits of cannabis while minimizing risks.

This chapter explores potential interactions between cannabis and medications, highlights

Cannabis for Chronic Pain: A Nutritionist's Guide to Relief

key nutritional factors to consider, and provides strategies for mitigating adverse effects and optimizing treatment outcomes. By combining research-based insights with practical applications, this chapter equips healthcare providers and patients with the knowledge needed for safe and effective integration of cannabis into a chronic pain management plan.

Cannabis for Chronic Pain: A Nutritionist's Guide to Relief

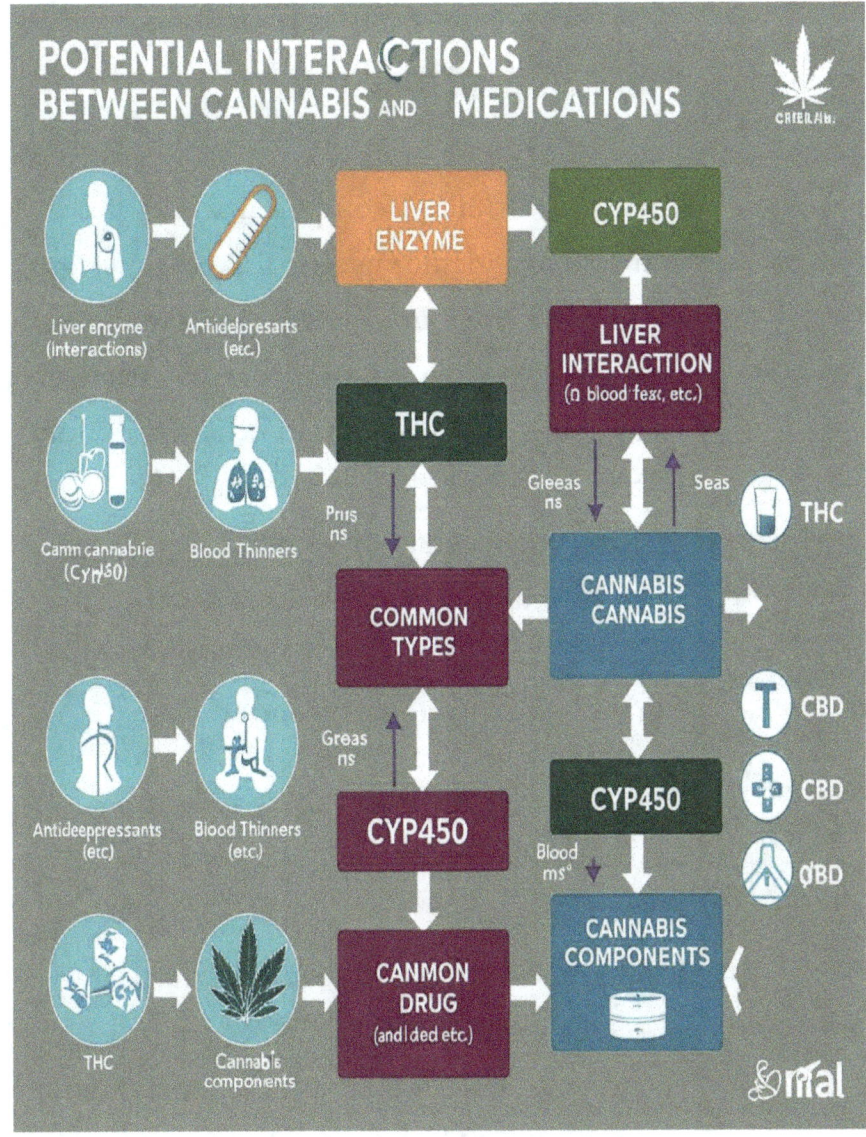

Cannabis and Medication Interactions

Cannabis for Chronic Pain: A Nutritionist's Guide to Relief

1. Potential Interactions Between Cannabis and Medications

Cannabis contains a complex mixture of active compounds, including cannabinoids such as tetrahydrocannabinol (THC) and cannabidiol (CBD). These compounds interact with the body primarily through the endocannabinoid system but also influence enzymes and receptors involved in drug metabolism. Understanding these interactions is critical for ensuring safety and efficacy when combining cannabis with other medications.

1.1. Role of Cytochrome P450 Enzymes

Cannabinoids are metabolized in the liver by the cytochrome P450 (CYP450) enzyme system, particularly by the enzymes CYP3A4 and CYP2C9. These enzymes also metabolize many common medications, leading to potential interactions.

- **Inhibition of CYP450 Enzymes**: CBD is a known inhibitor of CYP450 enzymes, which can slow the metabolism of certain drugs, increasing their blood levels and risk of side effects.
- **Induction of CYP450 Enzymes**: THC may induce some CYP450 enzymes, potentially lowering the efficacy of medications by speeding up their breakdown.

1.2. Common Medications Affected by Cannabis

- **Anticoagulants (e.g., Warfarin):** CBD can increase the effects of anticoagulants by inhibiting their metabolism, raising the risk of bleeding.

- **Antidepressants (e.g., SSRIs):** Cannabis may alter the metabolism of SSRIs, potentially leading to changes in efficacy or side effects like drowsiness or serotonin syndrome.

- **Antiepileptics (e.g., Clobazam):** CBD can increase the levels of clobazam and its active metabolite, heightening the risk of sedation and liver enzyme elevation.

- **Opioids**: Cannabis may enhance the pain-relieving effects of opioids but also increase the risk of respiratory depression and sedation.

- **Immunosuppressants (e.g., Tacrolimus):** THC and CBD may alter the metabolism of immunosuppressants, requiring dose adjustments to avoid toxicity or rejection of transplanted organs.

1.3. Risk Factors for Adverse Drug-Cannabis Interactions

Several factors influence the likelihood and severity of drug-cannabis interactions:

- **Dosage**: Higher doses of cannabinoids are more likely to cause significant interactions.
- **Age**: Older adults may have slower metabolism and increased sensitivity to drug interactions.
- **Liver Function**: Impaired liver function can exacerbate interactions by reducing the metabolism of both cannabinoids and medications.
- **Polypharmacy**: Individuals taking multiple medications are at greater risk of cumulative interactions.

2. Nutritional Considerations for Minimizing Adverse Effects

Cannabis for Chronic Pain: A Nutritionist's Guide to Relief

Nutrition plays a vital role in modulating the body's response to cannabis and medications. Certain dietary choices can mitigate side effects, enhance the body's ability to process cannabinoids, and improve overall treatment outcomes.

2.1. Enhancing Liver Function

The liver is central to metabolizing both cannabinoids and medications. Supporting liver health through nutrition can optimize metabolism and reduce the risk of adverse effects.

- **Foods Rich in Antioxidants:** Include berries, leafy greens, and citrus fruits to combat oxidative stress in the liver.
- **Cruciferous Vegetables**: Broccoli, kale, and Brussels sprouts can support liver enzyme function and detoxification.

Cannabis for Chronic Pain: A Nutritionist's Guide to Relief

- **Hydration**: Adequate water intake aids in flushing toxins and supporting metabolic processes.
- **Avoiding Excess Alcohol and Processed Foods:** These can impair liver function and exacerbate side effects.

2.2. Addressing Nutritional Deficiencies

Chronic pain patients often have nutritional deficiencies that can influence cannabis metabolism and effectiveness. Addressing these deficiencies is critical.

- **Magnesium**: Supports muscle relaxation and reduces the likelihood of cannabis-induced cramps or spasms. Found in nuts, seeds, and dark chocolate.
- **Vitamin D:** Plays a role in immune function and bone health. Low levels may exacerbate inflammation and pain.

- **B Vitamins**: Essential for nerve function and reducing the risk of neuropathic pain. Include whole grains, eggs, and fortified cereals.

2.3. Mitigating Side Effects of Cannabis

Cannabis use can cause side effects such as dry mouth, dizziness, and gastrointestinal discomfort. Nutritional strategies can help alleviate these issues.

- **Dry Mouth**: Increase water intake and consume hydrating foods like watermelon and cucumbers.
- **Dizziness**: Ensure adequate sodium and potassium intake, especially in individuals prone to low blood pressure.
- **Gastrointestinal Discomfort**: Include fiber-rich foods like oats and flaxseeds to support digestive health.

2.4. Timing Meals and Cannabis Use

The timing of meals can influence the absorption and effects of cannabis. Fat-soluble cannabinoids like THC and CBD are better absorbed when taken with a meal containing healthy fats.

- **Recommended Fats**: Avocado, olive oil, nuts, and fatty fish.
- **Avoid High-Sugar Foods**: These can cause blood sugar fluctuations, worsening side effects like dizziness or fatigue.

3. Strategies for Mitigating Potential Interactions

To minimize the risks of cannabis-medication and cannabis-nutrition interactions, a proactive approach is essential. These strategies combine clinical insights with practical recommendations for both healthcare providers and patients.

3.1. Collaborative Care

Healthcare providers should work together to ensure a comprehensive understanding of the patient's treatment plan.

- **Pharmacist Consultation**: Pharmacists can identify potential drug-cannabis interactions and recommend adjustments.
- **Dietitian Collaboration:** A dietitian can design a nutrition plan tailored to the individual's cannabis use and chronic pain needs.

3.2. Personalizing Cannabis Dosing

A personalized approach to cannabis dosing can minimize interactions and side effects:

- **Start Low, Go Slow**: Begin with a low dose of cannabis and gradually increase until therapeutic effects are achieved.
- **Microdosing**: Using small doses of cannabis may reduce the risk of interactions while providing symptom relief.

3.3. Regular Monitoring and Adjustments

Ongoing monitoring ensures that the treatment plan remains effective and safe.

- **Frequent Check-Ins:** Schedule regular appointments to assess efficacy and side effects.
- **Blood Tests**: Monitor liver enzymes and nutrient levels to identify potential issues early.

3.4. Education and Awareness

Educating patients about potential interactions and safe practices empowers them to make informed decisions.

- **Reading Labels**: Encourage patients to check product labels for CBD and THC concentrations.
- **Avoiding Grapefruit Juice**: Grapefruit juice can inhibit CYP450 enzymes, amplifying drug-cannabis interactions.
- **Being Transparent**: Patients should inform all healthcare providers about their cannabis use.

3.5. Alternative Therapies

In cases where cannabis-medication interactions pose significant risks, alternative therapies may be considered.

- **Topical Cannabis Products**: These have localized effects and are less likely to interact with systemic medications.
- **Non-Cannabinoid Pain Management**: Techniques such as acupuncture or physical therapy can complement or replace cannabis use.

Cannabis and nutrition offer promising avenues for chronic pain management, but their integration requires careful attention to potential interactions with medications and each other. By understanding the mechanisms of these interactions, addressing nutritional factors, and adopting proactive strategies, healthcare providers can help patients achieve effective and safe relief. Continuous monitoring, collaborative care, and patient

Cannabis for Chronic Pain: A Nutritionist's Guide to Relief

education are essential components of a successful plan that maximizes benefits while minimizing risks.

3.3: Overcoming Challenges and Staying Motivated: A Guide for Patients and Practitioners

Cannabis and nutrition therapy present a holistic approach to managing chronic pain. While the benefits can be transformative, implementing these therapies often comes with challenges. Patients may face physical, psychological, and social barriers, while practitioners might grapple with clinical uncertainties and patient adherence. Overcoming these obstacles is essential for long-term success.

This chapter identifies common challenges in cannabis and nutrition therapy for chronic pain, offers strategies to address these barriers, and highlights resources for ongoing support. Both patients and practitioners will gain

Cannabis for Chronic Pain: A Nutritionist's Guide to Relief
practical insights to stay motivated and navigate the complexities of personalized care.

1. Common Challenges in Cannabis and Nutrition Therapy

1.1. Challenges for Patients

1. Stigma Surrounding Cannabis Use
  - **Social Stigma**: Many patients face judgment from peers, family, or employers when using cannabis.
  - **Internalized Stigma**: Patients may feel guilty or hesitant about using cannabis despite its therapeutic potential.

2. Lack of Knowledge and Misinformation

Cannabis for Chronic Pain: A Nutritionist's Guide to Relief

- Patients may struggle to understand the complexities of cannabis and nutrition therapy due to conflicting information online and in the media.

- Misunderstandings about dosing, delivery methods, or potential side effects can lead to misuse or non-adherence.

3. Financial Barriers

- High costs of cannabis products, supplements, and specialized nutrition plans may deter long-term adherence.

- Lack of insurance coverage for cannabis-related treatments exacerbates financial strain.

4. Difficulty in Maintaining Dietary Changes

- Transitioning to a therapeutic diet can feel overwhelming, especially for individuals with limited cooking skills or busy schedules.

- Social and cultural influences on eating habits may conflict with prescribed nutrition plans.

5. Managing Expectations
- Some patients expect immediate relief and may feel discouraged when results take time.
- Unrealistic expectations about cannabis as a "cure-all" can lead to frustration and non-compliance.

1.2. Challenges for Practitioners

1. Navigating Legal and Regulatory Issues
- Practitioners must stay updated on rapidly evolving cannabis laws and regulations.
- Fear of professional repercussions may deter clinicians from recommending cannabis.

2. Limited Research and Evidence

Cannabis for Chronic Pain: A Nutritionist's Guide to Relief

- While evidence for cannabis in chronic pain is growing, gaps remain in understanding its long-term effects and interactions with specific dietary interventions.

- Practitioners may struggle to reconcile anecdotal patient reports with the available clinical evidence.

3. Patient Compliance and Communication

- Ensuring patients adhere to both cannabis regimens and nutritional plans can be challenging.

- Explaining complex concepts in an accessible way requires time and skill.

4. Personal Bias and Comfort Levels

- Some practitioners may feel uncomfortable recommending cannabis due to personal beliefs or lack of training.

- Bias against complementary therapies can hinder a fully integrated approach.

2. Strategies for Overcoming Challenges and Staying Motivated

2.1. For Patients

1. Education and Empowerment
   - **Seek Reliable Sources**: Use reputable organizations like the National Institute on Drug Abuse (NIDA) or the Academy of Nutrition and Dietetics.
   - **Work with Specialists**: Partner with certified cannabis practitioners and registered dietitians for tailored advice.
   - **Track Progress**: Keep a journal of symptoms, dietary intake, and cannabis use to monitor effectiveness.

Cannabis for Chronic Pain: A Nutritionist's Guide to Relief

2. Addressing Stigma

- **Open Communication**: Discuss concerns with trusted healthcare providers, family, and friends.

- **Advocacy**: Join support groups to connect with others navigating similar challenges.

3. Overcoming Financial Barriers

- **Explore Cost-Saving Options**: Consider generic cannabis products or government-approved programs for discounted access.

- **Prioritize Essentials**: Focus on core dietary changes and gradually incorporate supplements or premium products as budget allows.

4. Building Sustainable Habits

- **Start Small**: Make one or two dietary changes at a time rather than overhauling your entire routine.

- **Leverage Meal Prep**: Prepare meals in advance to save time and reduce stress.
- **Stay Flexible**: Adapt the plan to accommodate personal preferences and lifestyle changes.

5. Managing Expectations

- **Set Realistic Goals**: Understand that cannabis and nutrition therapy often yield gradual, not immediate, results.
- **Celebrate Progress:** Acknowledge even small improvements to stay motivated.

2.2. For Practitioners

1. Enhancing Knowledge and Skills

- **Continuing Education**: Attend cannabis and nutrition-focused conferences and workshops.

Cannabis for Chronic Pain: A Nutritionist's Guide to Relief

- **Stay Updated**: Follow journals such as The Journal of Pain and Nutrition Reviews for the latest research.

2. Navigating Legalities

- **Understand Local Laws**: Consult legal experts or professional organizations to stay compliant.
- **Document Decisions**: Maintain detailed patient records to protect against liability.

3. Improving Patient Engagement

- **Active Listening**: Build trust by addressing patient concerns and validating their experiences.
- **Simplify Instructions**: Provide clear, actionable steps rather than overwhelming patients with complex information.

4. Addressing Personal Bias

- **Reflect and Reevaluate**: Examine personal beliefs about cannabis and complementary therapies.

- **Collaborate with Colleagues**: Partner with practitioners who specialize in areas where you lack expertise.

3. Resources for Further Support and Guidance

3.1. For Patients

1. Educational Resources

- **Cannabis and Chronic Pain**: A Practical Guide: A patient-friendly book explaining cannabis use.

- **Nutrition.gov**: Provides evidence-based dietary advice and meal planning tools.

Cannabis for Chronic Pain: A Nutritionist's Guide to Relief

2. Support Groups

 - **Online Communities**: Forums like **Patients for Medical Cannabis** offer peer support and shared experiences.

 - **Local Meetups**: Many communities host in-person support groups for chronic pain patients.

3. Mobile Apps

 - **Cannabis Tracking**: Apps like **Releaf** help patients document cannabis use and symptoms.

 - **Nutrition Management**: Apps like **MyFitnessPal** assist with tracking dietary changes.

3.2. For Practitioners

1. Professional Organizations

- **Society of Cannabis Clinicians (SCC):** Offers education and networking opportunities.
- **Academy of Nutrition and Dietetics**: Provides tools for integrating nutrition into pain management.

2. Research Databases

- **PubMed**: Access to peer-reviewed articles on cannabis and nutrition.
- **Cannabis Science and Technology**: A journal focused on cannabis research and applications.

3. Clinical Tools

- **Dosing Calculators**: Online tools to estimate safe and effective cannabis dosages.
- **Dietary Assessment Platforms**: Software like **Nutritionist Pro** for creating customized nutrition plans.

Cannabis for Chronic Pain: A Nutritionist's Guide to Relief

Implementing cannabis and nutrition therapy for chronic pain is a multifaceted process that requires addressing various challenges. Patients and practitioners alike must stay informed, resilient, and collaborative to achieve long-term success. By leveraging educational resources, adopting strategic approaches, and fostering open communication, both groups can overcome obstacles and unlock the full potential of this integrative therapy. Staying motivated and committed to the process is key, as small steps forward can lead to significant improvements in quality of life.

Part 4: Case Studies and Future Directions

4.1: Real-Life Examples of Cannabis and Nutrition Therapy for Chronic Pain

Chronic pain is a complex condition that requires a multifaceted approach to management. Combining cannabis therapy with targeted nutritional strategies has emerged as a promising avenue for providing relief. In this chapter, we explore real-life case studies of individuals who have successfully utilized this integrative approach. Through these stories, we identify lessons learned and actionable insights that can guide patients and practitioners in implementing cannabis and nutrition therapies effectively.

Cannabis for Chronic Pain: A Nutritionist's Guide to Relief

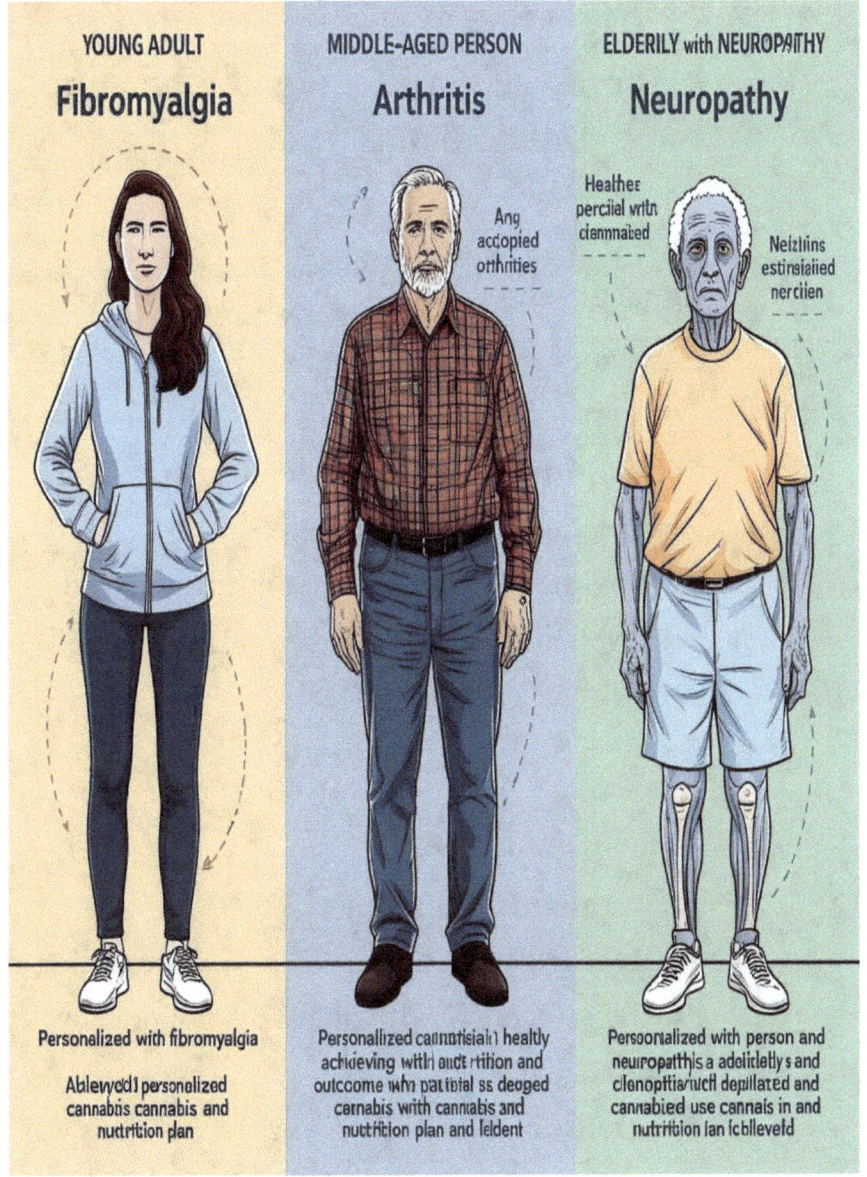

Patient Case Study Visualization

Cannabis for Chronic Pain: A Nutritionist's Guide to Relief

1. Case Study 1: Managing Fibromyalgia with Cannabis and an Anti-Inflammatory Diet

Background

- **Patient Profile**: Maria, a 42-year-old teacher diagnosed with fibromyalgia.
- **Symptoms**: Chronic widespread pain, fatigue, and sleep disturbances.
- **Previous Treatments**: Conventional pain relievers and physical therapy offered limited relief.

Intervention

1. Cannabis Regimen

  - **Dosage and Strain**: Maria was prescribed a low-THC, high-CBD oil taken sublingually twice daily.
  - **Delivery Method**: Vaporized cannabis was recommended for acute flare-ups.

Cannabis for Chronic Pain: A Nutritionist's Guide to Relief

2. Nutritional Plan

  - **Dietary Focus**: Anti-inflammatory diet emphasizing omega-3-rich foods, antioxidant-dense vegetables, and whole grains.

  - **Supplements**: Vitamin D and magnesium to address deficiencies.

Outcomes

- **Pain Levels**: Reported a 50% reduction in pain severity within three months.
- **Sleep Quality**: Improved sleep onset and reduced night awakenings.
- **Energy Levels**: Increased energy and reduced fatigue.

Key Takeaways

- **Synergy Between Cannabis and Nutrition:** The anti-inflammatory properties of cannabis complemented dietary efforts to reduce systemic inflammation.

- **Gradual Adjustments**: Starting with a low dose of cannabis minimized side effects and allowed Maria to build tolerance.

2. Case Study 2: Alleviating Osteoarthritis Pain with Cannabis and Collagen Supplementation

Background

- **Patient Profile**: John, a 67-year-old retired carpenter with osteoarthritis in the knees.
- **Symptoms**: Joint stiffness, swelling, and moderate pain interfering with mobility.
- **Previous Treatments**: NSAIDs and corticosteroid injections provided only temporary relief.

Cannabis for Chronic Pain: A Nutritionist's Guide to Relief

Intervention

1. Cannabis Regimen

 - **Dosage and Form**: Topical CBD cream applied to the knees twice daily, combined with oral THC/CBD capsules (1:1 ratio) taken at bedtime.

2. Nutritional Plan

 - **Dietary Adjustments**: Increased intake of bone broth and collagen-rich foods to support joint health.

 - **Weight Management**: Implemented a calorie-controlled Mediterranean diet to reduce excess weight burdening the joints.

Outcomes

- **Pain Reduction**: Significant decrease in joint pain within six weeks.

Cannabis for Chronic Pain: A Nutritionist's Guide to Relief

- **Mobility**: Improved range of motion and reduced morning stiffness.
- **Inflammation**: Marked decrease in knee swelling, as evidenced by physical exams.

Key Takeaways

- **Localized Relief**: Topical CBD provided targeted pain relief without systemic side effects.
- **Joint Health Focus**: Collagen supplementation complemented the anti-inflammatory effects of cannabis.

3. Case Study 3: Treating Migraine Pain with Cannabis and Magnesium Optimization

Cannabis for Chronic Pain: A Nutritionist's Guide to Relief

Background

- **Patient Profile**: Rachel, a 29-year-old software engineer with chronic migraines.
- **Symptoms**: Intense headache episodes occurring 10–15 days per month, often accompanied by nausea and sensitivity to light.
- **Previous Treatments**: Prescription triptans and beta-blockers provided inconsistent relief.

Intervention

1. Cannabis Regimen

   - **Delivery Method**: Rachel used a CBD-rich tincture daily and vaporized THC during acute migraine attacks.

2. Nutritional Plan

   - **Magnesium Supplementation**: Introduced 400 mg of magnesium glycinate daily.
   - **Dietary Changes**: Avoided migraine triggers, such as processed meats and artificial

sweeteners, while increasing magnesium-rich foods like leafy greens, nuts, and seeds.

Outcomes

- **Frequency**: Migraine days reduced by 60% after three months.
- **Intensity**: Decreased severity of remaining migraines.
- **Nausea**: Improved tolerance to light and sound during migraine episodes.

Key Takeaways

- **Magnesium Synergy:** Optimized magnesium levels enhanced the efficacy of cannabis in reducing migraine frequency.
- **Trigger Identification**: Avoiding dietary triggers played a crucial role in overall symptom management.

4. Lessons Learned from Case Studies

1. Personalized Approaches Are Essential
 - Tailored cannabis regimens and **nutritional** plans are critical for addressing individual needs and responses.

2. Cannabis Delivery Methods Matter
 - The choice between oral, topical, and inhaled cannabis impacts effectiveness and patient adherence.

3. Dietary Changes Enhance Cannabis Efficacy
 - Nutritional strategies targeting inflammation, deficiencies, or triggers amplify cannabis's therapeutic potential.

4. Long-Term Commitment

- Success often requires patience, regular monitoring, and adjustments to the plan based on progress.

5. Interdisciplinary Collaboration
  - Combining expertise from cannabis specialists, dietitians, and primary care providers ensures a comprehensive approach.

5. Practical Applications for Patients and Practitioners

For Patients

- **Keep a Symptom Journal**: Track cannabis use, dietary changes, and symptom patterns to identify what works best.

- **Communicate with Healthcare Providers**: Share progress and challenges openly for more effective care.

For Practitioners

- **Educate Patients**: Provide clear instructions on dosing, delivery methods, and dietary interventions.
- **Stay Updated**: Incorporate the latest research on cannabis and nutrition into practice.

Real-life examples illustrate the transformative potential of integrating cannabis and nutrition therapy for chronic pain. These case studies highlight the importance of personalization, patient education, and ongoing monitoring to achieve optimal outcomes. As evidence continues to grow, these approaches will likely become increasingly central to chronic pain management strategies. By learning from past successes and challenges, patients and

Cannabis for Chronic Pain: A Nutritionist's Guide to Relief

practitioners can work together to create effective, sustainable treatment plans.

4.2: The Future of Cannabis and Nutrition Research: Emerging Trends and Opportunities

The intersection of cannabis and nutrition represents a promising frontier in chronic pain management. While existing research has established foundational insights, significant gaps remain in our understanding of the synergistic effects between these two therapeutic modalities. As cannabis becomes increasingly accepted in medical practice and nutrition's role in health continues to be emphasized, the need for robust, evidence-based research grows. This chapter explores current research gaps, emerging trends, and future opportunities in the field, along with their implications for clinical practice and patient care.

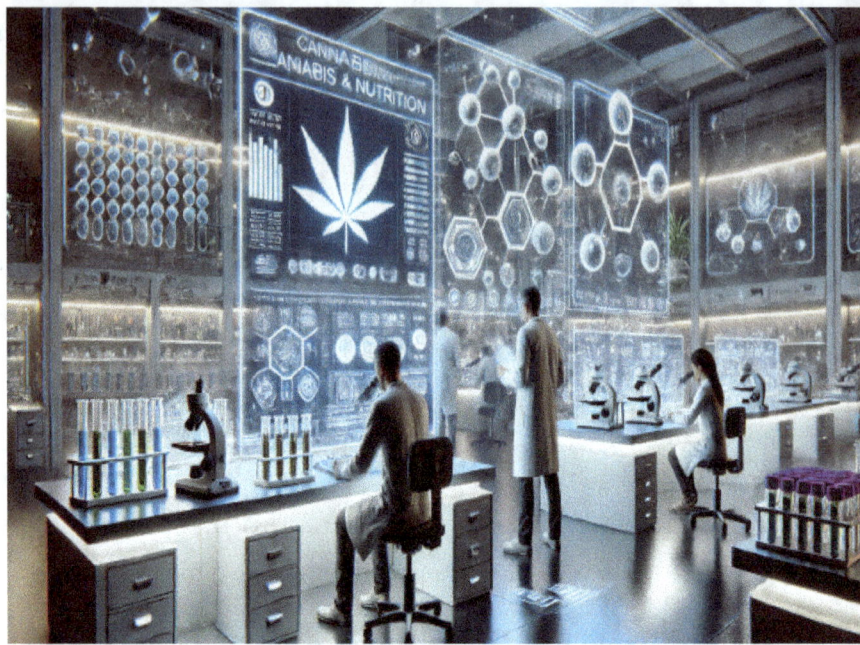

The Future of Cannabis and Nutrition Research

1. Overview of Current Research Gaps

1.1. Lack of Large-Scale, Longitudinal Studies
- **Problem**: Most studies on cannabis and nutrition are small-scale and short-term, limiting generalizability.

- **Impact**: A lack of long-term data on safety, efficacy, and side effects inhibits the development of standardized treatment protocols.
- **Example**: Limited understanding of how chronic cannabis use interacts with long-term dietary patterns in pain management.

1.2. Insufficient Focus on Individual Variability

- **Genetic Factors**: How genetic polymorphisms in the endocannabinoid system (e.g., CB1 and CB2 receptors) affect responses to cannabis.
- **Dietary Influences**: Variability in nutritional status (e.g., deficiencies in omega-3 or magnesium) and its impact on cannabis efficacy.
- **Patient-Specific Outcomes**: Need for personalized treatment plans based on age, gender, weight, and metabolic health.

1.3. Interactions Between Cannabis and Nutrients

- **Gap**: Limited understanding of how specific nutrients, such as vitamins, minerals, and phytonutrients, interact with cannabis to influence bioavailability and therapeutic effects.
- **Example**: Potential for omega-3 fatty acids to enhance endocannabinoid signaling remains underexplored.

1.4. Limited Research on Special Populations

- **Pregnancy and Lactation**: Lack of data on the safety of cannabis and nutrition interventions during these stages.
- **Elderly Populations**: Unique metabolic considerations in aging individuals with chronic pain.

2. Emerging Trends in Cannabis and Nutrition Research

2.1. Integration of Personalized Medicine

- **Advances in Genomics**: Growing use of genetic testing to identify individual variations in cannabinoid receptor expression and nutritional needs.
- **Personalized Diets**: Tailoring dietary recommendations to complement cannabis therapy for specific conditions like arthritis, migraines, or neuropathy.

2.2. The Role of the Microbiome

- **Gut-Cannabinoid Axis**: Emerging research suggests a bidirectional relationship between the gut microbiome and the endocannabinoid system.

- **Example**: Certain gut bacteria may modulate the effects of cannabis on inflammation and pain.
- **Probiotic and Prebiotic Synergy**: Investigating how dietary interventions to support the microbiome can enhance cannabis's therapeutic potential.

2.3. Advances in Cannabinoid Delivery Systems

- **Nanotechnology**: Development of nanoparticles to improve cannabinoid bioavailability and absorption.
- **Encapsulation Methods**: Combining cannabis with lipid-based carriers to enhance delivery through the digestive system.
- **Fortified Foods**: Exploring the potential of cannabinoid-infused functional foods designed for pain relief.

2.4. Exploration of Terpenes and Flavonoids

- **Terpene Effects**: Investigating how compounds like myrcene, limonene, and beta-caryophyllene contribute to pain relief and interact with dietary components.
- **Flavonoids in Nutrition**: Synergistic effects of flavonoid-rich foods (e.g., berries, dark chocolate) with cannabis compounds.

2.5. Multi-Modal Therapies

- **Combination Approaches**: Integrating cannabis, nutrition, physical therapy, and mindfulness techniques for holistic pain management.
- **Case Study Programs**: Real-world applications of these combinations in clinical settings.

3. Opportunities in Cannabis and Nutrition Research

3.1. Cross-Disciplinary Collaborations

- **Collaboration Between Disciplines**: Partnerships between cannabis researchers, nutritionists, and clinicians to design comprehensive studies.
- **Industry Involvement**: Engaging cannabis and nutritional supplement companies in funding innovative research.

3.2. Use of Artificial Intelligence (AI) and Machine Learning

- **Predictive Analytics**: Leveraging AI to identify patterns in patient responses to cannabis and nutrition interventions.
- **Data Integration**: Using AI to analyze large datasets from wearable devices, patient reports, and clinical trials.

3.3. Expanding the Scope of Cannabinoid Research

- **Minor Cannabinoids**: Investigating the therapeutic roles of lesser-known cannabinoids, such as CBG, CBC, and THCV.
- **Plant-Based Diets and Cannabinoids**: Examining how vegan or vegetarian diets affect cannabinoid metabolism.

3.4. Ethical and Regulatory Considerations

- **Ethical Studies**: Conducting research with rigorous ethical oversight, especially in vulnerable populations.
- **Policy Advocacy:** Promoting evidence-based policies to support cannabis and nutrition research.

4. Implications for Clinical Practice and Patient Care

4.1. Enhanced Patient Education

- **Interactive Tools**: Development of apps and digital platforms to educate patients about the interaction between cannabis and nutrition.
- **Tailored Guidance**: Providing personalized recommendations based on the latest research.

4.2. Evidence-Based Protocols

- **Standardized Guidelines**: Establishing clinical protocols for integrating cannabis and nutrition in chronic pain management.
- **Ongoing Training**: Offering continuing education for practitioners to stay updated on emerging trends.

4.3. Focus on Holistic Care

- **Patient-Centered Approaches**: Emphasizing the importance of lifestyle factors, including diet, exercise, and mental health, in conjunction with cannabis therapy.

- **Collaborative Care Models**: Encouraging interdisciplinary teams to address complex chronic pain cases.

The future of cannabis and nutrition research is rich with potential to transform chronic pain management. Addressing current gaps in research, embracing emerging trends, and fostering interdisciplinary collaborations will be critical in advancing this field. For practitioners, integrating these insights into clinical practice can provide patients with more effective, personalized, and holistic care. As the scientific community continues to explore the synergistic effects of cannabis and nutrition, the opportunities for innovation and improved patient outcomes are boundless.

4.3: Conclusion and Final Thoughts

The journey through **Cannabis for Chronic Pain: A Nutritionist's Guide to Relief** has provided a comprehensive understanding of how cannabis and nutrition, as complementary therapies, can transform the management of chronic pain. By delving into the science, practical applications, and real-world case studies, this book has sought to empower both practitioners and patients with knowledge and tools to navigate this promising but evolving landscape.

In this concluding chapter, we will revisit the key takeaways, reflect on the potential of cannabis and nutrition therapy, and encourage further exploration into this integrative approach to pain relief.

Cannabis for Chronic Pain: A Nutritionist's Guide to Relief

1. Recap of Key Takeaways

1.1. The Science Behind Cannabis and Pain Management

- **Endocannabinoid System (ECS):** Central to cannabis's therapeutic effects, the ECS plays a crucial role in regulating pain, inflammation, and homeostasis.

- **Cannabinoids in Pain Relief**: Key compounds like THC and CBD offer anti-inflammatory, analgesic, and neuroprotective properties.

- **Synergistic Effects**: Cannabis compounds work together in the "entourage effect," amplifying therapeutic outcomes.

Cannabis for Chronic Pain: A Nutritionist's Guide to Relief

1.2. Nutrition's Role in Chronic Pain Management

- **Anti-Inflammatory Diets**: Diets rich in omega-3 fatty acids, antioxidants, and phytochemicals reduce systemic inflammation and pain.

- **Micronutrient Balance**: Magnesium, vitamin D, and other essential nutrients support muscle relaxation, nerve function, and ECS modulation.

- **Gut Health**: The gut microbiome influences inflammation and interacts with the ECS, underscoring the importance of prebiotics, probiotics, and fiber.

1.3. Cannabis and Nutrition: A Synergistic Approach

- **Enhancing Cannabis Efficacy**: Nutritional strategies can optimize cannabinoid absorption and bioavailability, improving therapeutic outcomes.

- **Personalized Plans:** Integrating dietary and cannabis interventions tailored to individual needs ensures more effective pain management.

1.4. Practical Strategies for Implementation

- **Assessment and Planning:** Evaluating individual needs, setting realistic goals, and monitoring progress are essential for successful therapy.
- **Addressing Challenges**: Overcoming stigma, navigating legal complexities, and managing potential interactions require informed decision-making and support.
- **Holistic Integration**: Combining cannabis and nutrition with lifestyle modifications, such as exercise and mindfulness, enhances overall well-being.

2. Final Thoughts on the Potential of Cannabis and Nutrition Therapy

2.1. A Paradigm Shift in Chronic Pain Management

- **Beyond Symptom Relief**: Cannabis and nutrition therapies address underlying causes of chronic pain, offering sustainable, long-term solutions.

- **Patient Empowerment:** This integrative approach shifts the focus from passive treatment to active participation in health management.

2.2. Bridging the Gaps in Knowledge and Access

- **Education and Awareness**: Expanding public and professional knowledge about cannabis and nutrition is critical to breaking down stigma and misinformation.

- **Research Imperatives**: Continued investment in rigorous scientific studies will refine our understanding of these therapies and their combined potential.
- **Access and Equity**: Efforts to make cannabis and nutrition therapies accessible to diverse populations are vital for inclusive care.

2.3. Holistic Care for Complex Conditions

- **Interdisciplinary Collaboration:** Nutritionists, medical professionals, and cannabis specialists working together can create comprehensive care plans.
- **Mental Health Integration**: Recognizing the psychological impact of chronic pain, this approach supports mental and emotional resilience.

3. Encouragement for Further Exploration and Discovery

3.1. For Practitioners

- **Stay Informed**: Keeping abreast of emerging research and clinical practices ensures the delivery of cutting-edge care.
- **Advocate for Patients**: Champion the inclusion of cannabis and nutrition in mainstream medical discussions and policies.
- **Collaborate and Share Knowledge**: Building networks with peers in related fields fosters innovation and improves patient outcomes.

3.2. For Patients

- **Be Open to New Possibilities**: Exploring integrative therapies can uncover new paths to relief and empowerment.

- **Seek Expert Guidance**: Working with qualified professionals ensures safe and effective use of cannabis and nutrition therapies.
- **Take an Active Role**: Engaging in your care plan through informed decisions and consistent effort enhances success.

3.3. For Researchers and Innovators

- **Investigate Uncharted Areas**: Focus on underexplored topics, such as cannabis-nutrition interactions and patient-specific outcomes.
- **Develop Tools and Resources**: Create accessible technologies and educational materials to support practitioners and patients.
- **Champion Ethical Practices**: Ensure that research and innovation prioritize safety, efficacy, and inclusivity.

4. Practical Implications and Vision for the Future

4.1. Building Comprehensive Care Models

- **Integration in Healthcare**: Cannabis and nutrition therapies should become integral components of pain management protocols.
- **Tailored Solutions**: Personalization based on genetics, lifestyle, and health status will define future care strategies.

4.2. A Sustainable Approach to Health

- **Reducing Dependence on Pharmaceuticals**: By addressing pain through natural and dietary interventions, we can minimize reliance on medications with severe side effects.
- **Promoting Preventive Health**: Educating patients about nutrition and cannabis can

prevent chronic pain conditions from developing.

4.3. Expanding the Therapeutic Toolbox

- **Holistic Modalities**: Incorporating cannabis and nutrition with acupuncture, physical therapy, and stress management will redefine chronic pain care.
- **Global Opportunities**: Leveraging this knowledge across cultures and regions can democratize access to innovative therapies.

The synthesis of cannabis and nutrition represents a transformative opportunity in the fight against chronic pain. By combining scientific evidence with personalized care, this integrative approach offers a path to not only alleviate suffering but also empower patients to reclaim their lives. As the field continues to grow, collaboration among practitioners, researchers, and policymakers will be essential to unlocking its full potential.

This book is not the end but a starting point—an invitation to explore, innovate, and refine the art and science of cannabis and nutrition therapy. Together, we can turn the promise of these therapies into a reality for millions affected by chronic pain, fostering a future where relief is accessible, personalized, and enduring.

Cannabis for Chronic Pain: A Nutritionist's Guide to Relief

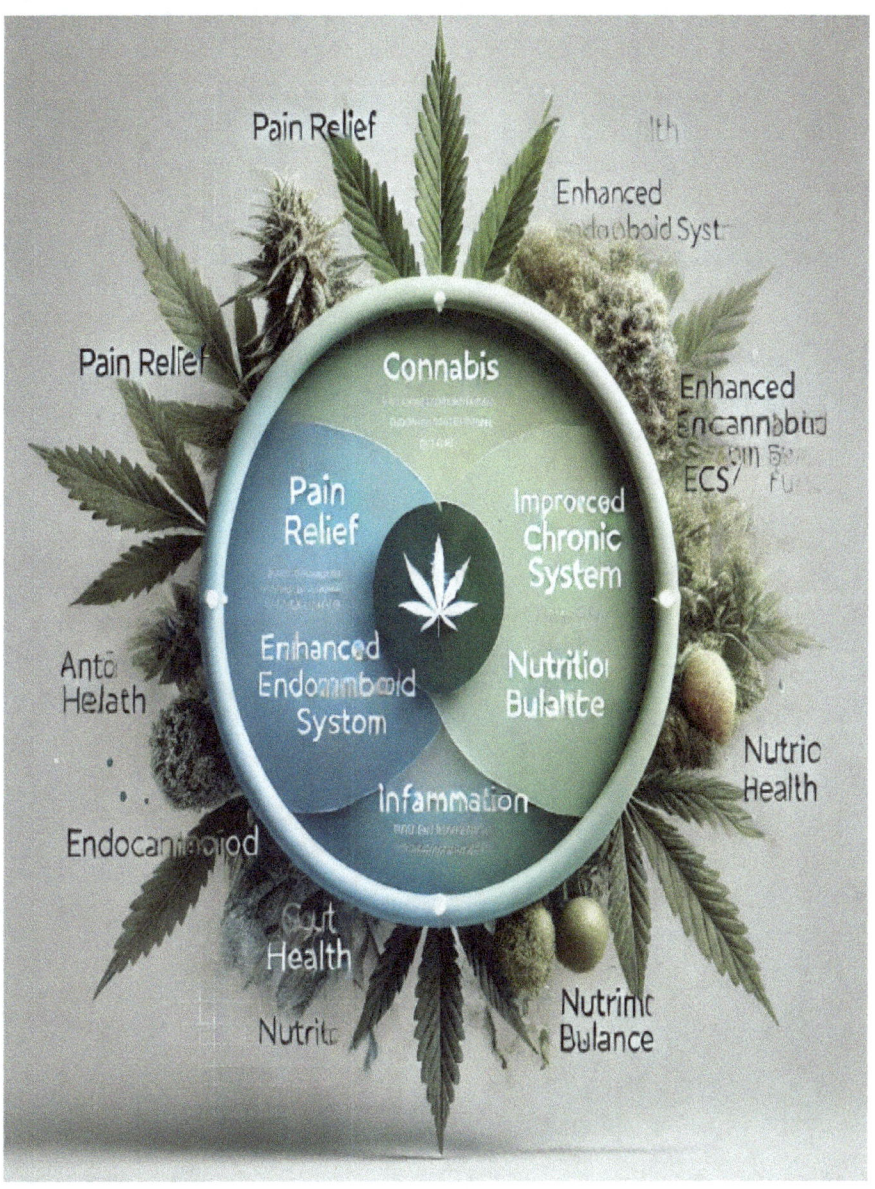

Cannabis-Nutrition Synergy Summary

www.ingramcontent.com/pod-product-compliance
Lightning Source LLC
Chambersburg PA
CBHW070954240526
45469CB00016B/811